PREGNANCY A.
YEARS OF YOUR CHILD'S LIFE
FROM 0 TO 5

Complete Health Guide
for Moms and Dads

MARY SIMMONS

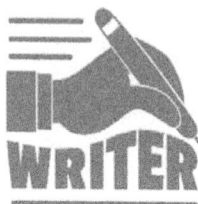

Here's your bonus

http://marysimmonsbook.com/home/

Table of Contents

FOREWORD

I feel greatly honored to have been given the privilege to write this foreword for Mary Simmons' new educational book. This feeling of mine is basically for two reasons. The first is that I know Mary Simmons personally while the second reason is that I am confident about the quality of the content of this book after reading through it. Mary Simmons has proven to be a loyal and good friend over the years which gives me a solid foundation to comment about her personality.

Her commitment to providing quality materials radiates throughout this book. Having read it, what I can say unflinchingly is that it is thoroughly researched and meticulously written to ensure that it is is based on fact and not sentiments or conjectures. The book reflects objectivity and a desire to provide people with a solid truth value.

This book was written to provide people with contents that will improve the quality of their lives. It is a complete guide that will help various people such as pregnant women, nursing mothers, expectant fathers as well as parents who are raising kids. The book provides a step-by-step guide concerning every subject in the book which is all concerned with improving the experience of the readers. Generally, the book is a complete package for a healthy and happy family.

This book will be a great help to parents-to-be who want to take care of their newborn babies and understand the process to the core. The information was constructed to provide readers with valuable and meaningful information. Normally, it would have been easy to get bored when reading this kind of book but Mary Simmons displays excellent writing acumen that makes the book fascinating and compelling – it keeps you on your toes all the way.

What you have in your hand is an educational and enterprising book capable of transforming your life incredibly. I will advise you not to read the book casually but with the intention of improving your experience as a person. By the time you are done reading the book, I am confident that you will gladly recommend it to your friends, families, and colleagues. The book is a worthwhile gift for people who matter to you. Get ready to be exposed to a simplified version of many concepts that used to sound complex. You are about to embark on a journey that will radically change your life. Cherish it, value it!

Stanley Cordar

INTRODUCTION

The important things in life are not necessarily complex things but simple things that have to be handled well. This book is a product of days and night of thorough research to provide you with material that is capable of adding value to your life. This is not your typical science-oriented book in spite of the fact that it contains a lot of scientific information. Every concept is dutifully and vividly explained such that you don't need to have a solid science background to comprehend the content of this book.

Parenting is full of both good and bad times. There will be ups and downs. However, you can reduce the bad days during various phases of childbearing and child raising by paying attention to details. Your life is a blank sheet where you write a new chapter daily. You have the right to choose to write memorable and lovely experiences daily or fill your life with unpleasant events day in, day out.

It is true that life will test you with various circumstances that will require you to be strong, but you have a huge part to play in your experiences in life. An important way to improve your experience in life is by reading quality books that can add value to your life. The fact that you have made a commitment to read this book shows that you are ready to improve your life by acquiring the requisite knowledge for a life with less stress and more fulfilling moments.

This book will help you have a better understanding of everything you need to know while waiting for a child and while raising your child. When you are well informed, you will not live life by chance. A trial and error approach to life is not profitable to you because you can lose irreplaceable things or even people. This material was written with the intent of helping people have happy homes and experiencing fewer issues when expecting a child or showing a child the ropes in life.

What you have at your disposal is a book that has tips that can revolutionize your approach to the way you handle your kids. You will understand your child much more and will be able to train them to have the bright future you intend for them.

You will be able to raise healthy kids because of the quality of information you will receive in this book. Pay attention to every piece of information you read in this book because they are treasures that will guide you on your way to successful parenting. Fasten your seat belt and enjoy this awesome and educational ride!

Part One

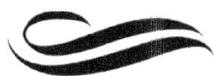

PARENTAL EDUCATION

This part introduces you to important components of parental education that you need to get a good grasp of as a parent. The information contained in this part will set you on a course of being empowered to take good care of yourself before getting married, during pregnancy, and after you deliver the baby.

This should not in any way put you off as a male because there are important things you also need to learn in order to be a quality partner for your wife all through these phases. Pay attention and learn as much as you can, because the information you are about to be exposed to is important in ensuring that your family stays healthy and happy.

BEFORE GETTING PREGNANT

A pregnancy, especially for a newly-wedded couple, is a wonderful thing. Things get better when they have been waiting for the fruit of the womb for a while. The happiness can be indescribable! However, there are some important things you need to know and put in place before you get pregnant. Some of these important tips are discussed below:

Avoid smoking

You have probably heard this statement more than a thousand time before now. When something true is repeated consistently, there is a tendency for you to see it as a cliché. However, you cannot afford to treat this important instruction as a cliché because it is not. Smoking is not just injurious to you, it is also harmful to your unborn child. The Better Health Channel suggests that merely breathing the smoke from someone else's cigarette, or second-hand smoke, is harmful to your health.

Watch out for Vitamin A

Vitamin A is good for your body because it is good for your vision and helps improve the performance of your immune system. It would be ridiculous to suggest that you should avoid Vitamin A. However, you need to be careful with the amount you consume when trying to get pregnant. The reason for this is that excess Vitamin A can lead to birth defects. It is safe if you don't consume more than the recommended 770 mcg RAE daily. Talk to your doctor if you are not sure about the supplement that is best for you.

Reduce your caffeine consumption

Caffeine is present in several everyday products such as soft drinks and beverages. However, for the sake of yourself and your child, you need to cut down your daily caffeine intake. In the NSW Mothersafe Handout for pregnant women, it is recommended that a pregnant woman not take more than 200mg of caffeine daily. In case you are wondering how you will be able to know that you are not taking beyond 200mg, it is pretty simple. Simply ensure that you don't take more than one strong espresso, four cups of instant coffee, or three cups of brewed coffee in a day.

More folic acid

It will help to take more folic acid as you prepare to get pregnant. Folic acid is important because it can affect the neural tube of your baby. The Centers for Disease Control and Prevention (CDC) posits that your child has a 50%-70% chance of not being affected by neural tube defects when you take 400mg of folic acid daily. Apart from this, there are also other birth-related defects that can be avoided when you make a practice of consuming folic acid every day.

Avoid drinking alcohol

Some researchers have identified the consumption of alcohol as one of the factors that affect fertility. Interestingly, it is not only women whose fertility is affected, but also men. Heavy drinking affects the sex drive of men and can also make them impotent. According to research co-authored by Boston University School of Public Health in 2016, it was observed that heavy drinking reduces the chances of getting pregnant for women. Hence, it is recommended that both you and your partner stay off alcohol as much as possible to increase your chance of having a baby.

Eat a balanced diet

This is another statement you will have heard a lot of times. A balanced diet is a meal that contains all the classes of food in the proper proportion. Such meals will nourish your body and prepare it to nurture a child. Malnourishing your body can affect your fertility or even impair your child when you eventually get pregnant. You should to cut down on junk food and eat well.

Make your fitness your priority

Don't misunderstand this. I am not talking about weight loss. You don't have to necessarily lose weight to look healthy but good fitness will help prepare your body for the rigors associated with labor. Your rate of recovery after delivery will also be faster if you are healthy and fit before getting pregnant. It helps to exercise regularly to put your body in the proper shape to receive a child. This will have both short-term and long-term benefits.

Go for genetic carrier screening

The essence of a genetic carrier screening is to help you and your partner find out if you have any critical conditions that might have been passed on to either of you by your parents, such as sickle cell disease and cystic fibrosis. These can be passed on to your child if care is not taken. You will be informed of the reproductive decisions you need to make in this case. The amazing thing about this screening is that it is very simple because you only need to provide a blood sample or saliva.

Go for a cervical screening test

Another screening test you can consider is a cervical screening test. It is not advisable to have this test regularly because it can affect your body negatively. It is better to do it no more than once every three years. It is also not advisable to do while pregnant. The essence of this test is to help you find out if your cervix has any unusual cells, which have the tendency to cause cervical cancer.

Ensure you have received the MMR vaccination

The MMR vaccination (measles, mumps and rubella) is usually administered to children before they are six years old. You need to verify whether you have been given this vaccination before you get pregnant, primarily because of rubella. Rubella is not common but can affect the development of your child negatively if you have it. Therefore, you need to make sure you know if you have been vaccinated.

DURING PREGNANCY

Pregnancy is a sensitive state for a woman. Any health issues during this time will not only affect the mother, but also the child. It is important that you pay attention and get any help you need so that you can have a successful delivery and a healthy child. There are some important things you need to consider when you are pregnant. Some of them are highlighted for you here:

Don't announce hastily

I know that feeling! You are so excited that you are going to be a mother. It is natural to be tempted to put it on your social media so that your friends can celebrate with you. But it is better to tell only members of your family until after you are three months along. No one wants anything to happen to their baby, but the truth is that it is especially vulnerable in the first trimester. Should anything tragic happen, you don't want to find yourself in the position of having to explain it over and over.

Be disciplined with your diet

During pregnancy, it is especially important to be disciplined with your diet for the sake of your health and that of your baby. There are some foods you need to avoid because they may end up being injurious to your health and the delivery process. Foods like beef and seafood such as mussels and oysters, if they are not properly cooked have the tendency to carry diseases like salmonella or toxoplasmosis. Salmonella infects the small intestine while toxoplasmosis can affect your brain, heart, eyes, and lungs. These diseases can be passed on to your baby. Caution is necessary.

Avoid exposure to toxicity

The last thing you want to do as a pregnant woman is to allow toxic substances from the environment to get into your system. This can occur even through such innocent activities as painting the nursery! Paints contain a level of toxicity that is not tolerable for a pregnant woman. It is better to ask someone else to paint the nursery for you rather than to expose yourself.

Don't be careless with your medications

Some medications are not good for pregnant women. You cannot afford to be careless during this period. You should look at your medication bottles to see if they have warnings for pregnant women. You should also check with your doctor to be sure that the medications that were prescribed to you before you got pregnant are still safe. A drug like Ibuprofen, for example, should be avoided because it can affect your baby. You have a higher chance of having a miscarriage if you take Ibuprofen regularly. It is safer to take Tylenol if you need a painkiller during pregnancy. But it's always better to talk to your doctor first.

Cut down your intake of caffeine

You need to cut down on your intake of caffeine before you get pregnant, but it is much more important after you become pregnant. As a stimulant, caffeine increases the rate at which your heart beats and also raises your blood pressure. Your metabolism can handle caffeine, but your baby's cannot. Unfortunately, caffeine moves into the body of your baby from you through the placenta. So the more you reduce your intake of caffeine during pregnancy, the better for you and your baby. A range of 150mg to 300mg is recommended.

Use caution when wearing heels

Heels are a popular fashion statement, but you need to take caution with them when you are pregnant. Your priority during this time should not be beauty, but the health of your baby. The more your stomach enlarges, the harder it will be for you to maintain your footing when walking. In order to avoid falling down, it is better to wear heels that are three inches high or less. You can rock any heel you want after delivering your baby.

Make use of lotions frequently

This is more for your benefit than the baby's. During your first pregnancy, it is likely that things will be a little rougher than in subsequent pregnancies. For example, you may develop stretch marks all over your body. You can prepare for this change by using lotion frequently. Your body does not have to become unrecognizable because of pregnancy. You can still look attractive in spite of the protrusion of your belly.

Do helpful exercises

The general rule during pregnancy is to avoid straining yourself unnecessarily to help prevent miscarriage or harming your unborn child. However, a moderate workout out plan is still recommended. You have to take care of yourself, but that does not mean that you should become lazy. Little exercises here and there will keep you fit and ready for the rigors of labor. It is important to talk to your doctor about your exercise plan so that you don't overexert yourself.

Avoid using the hot tub as much as possible

It is very tempting at times to relax in a hot tub. However, it is healthier to stay away from them while pregnant. The high heat is not healthy for your child and can cause some birth defects. If you are uncomfortable and craving relaxation, have a warm bath, but resist the higher temperature of the hot tub.

Get maternity clothes

This is quite obvious but it is very important. You need to get maternity clothes as you await the delivery of your little one. Remember that you will not need them for long, and you will have other expenses as well, so it is pointless to spend a lot of money, but you will want to be as comfortable as possible.

RELATIONSHIPS IN THE FAMILY

We are made for one another. Our relationships are the most important things in life, and the connection that exists among members of a family is vital because the home is the first training center for a child. It is the first school the child attends and it forms the core fabric of the value system of the society. Here are some tips that can help you maintain a happy home during this time of change and afterward:

Value the relationship more than material things

The family is not a business enterprise. It is a place where core values such as sharing, selflessness, and forgiveness are held in high esteem. There is a high rate of family breakups through divorce these days. Many of those breakups could have been avoided if people treated their family not as an avenue to enrich themselves and get what they want, but a platform to help one another grow.

It is wrong to treat members of your family less than they deserve simply because they are not as rich as you would have wanted. You need to value your husband in spite of how much he is making because bad times don't last forever. Learn to value what brought you together more than what he owns or does not own. Material things will come and go; family is forever.

Be a friend all the way

Things will not always go as planned for you and your family. Tough times don't change people, but they do reveal your true character. Members of your family need you the most during their down periods. Your husband needs you most when things are tough for him. Your kids need you the most when other people are treating them with less respect because of their failings.

Let members of your family remember you as a friend who stood by them through thick and thin. They may not say much at the moment. But one thing is sure: you will have written your name in gold on their hearts for the rest of their lives. They will see you as an example of motherhood and an embodiment of what a quality wife should look like. Anybody can stick around during the good times; only true friends stick around during tough periods.

Forgive in advance

Most times, we find it easier to forgive people who are not close to us, as opposed to people who are close to us. The reason for this is not far-fetched. The issue is that you expect people who are not close to you to hurt you. So, when they hurt you eventually, you are not too surprised and easily find a place in your heart to forgive them especially when they apologize. There is the likelihood that you will not apply the same rule for members of your family.

You are likely to assume that members of your family will not hurt you. Then, when they do, you find it a pill too bitter to swallow. You begin to wonder what you have done to them to deserve such unfair treatment. As wrong as it is for members of your family to hurt you, it is worse for you to assume that they cannot. That does not mean that you should go around waiting for them to hurt you, but the truth is that they most likely will at one point or another.

The earlier you accept that fact, the better. When you accept that they can hurt you, you will find it easier to forgive them. The best form of forgiveness that can be practiced in a happy home is what I call advance forgiveness. What this means is that you should learn to forgive members of your family long before they've even committed any wrong against you. This approach will strengthen the family and make it a fortress too difficult to invade by outsiders.

Keep your secrets safe with one another

A family that does not have the culture of keeping their secrets safe with one another is a ticking time bomb. Not everything that goes on in your family should be revealed to outsiders. In this era of social media, you need to be much more careful. It is safer to consult members of your family before you put things that have to do with them online.

They might end up seeing it as a betrayal of trust which will hurt them more than you can imagine. Don't be quick to share information about events in your family with the public because you might be digging the grave of the happiness that exists in your family. Place value on members of your family; keep their secrets safe.

Have respect for the opinion of others

Your family will not benefit from an attitude where you only listen to your own voice. Even if you are going to dismiss the opinion of others when making family decisions, it must be done in a way where the other person understands why you are doing it, and that it is not because you don't value his or her opinion. It must be clear from the way you speak that their opinion also counts but a decision that is best for all has to be made.

You will be making room for strive and hate when it is apparent to members of your family that they have no say in family decisions. Relationships in the family do not have to be toxic. A good way to go about this is by providing opportunities for others to say their mind while you objectively reach a consensus together.

WHAT MOTHERS SHOULD EXPECT WHEN THEY ARE EXPECTING

There is no argument about the fact that motherhood is a noble profession. You probably watched your mother with keen interest when you were younger. You probably wondered what was going through her head if she was expecting a new baby. Now it is your turn! There are things you should expect as a woman who is expecting a child. I have gathered some of the most important topics below for your perusal:

A desire to search the internet often

As a mother-to-be, you will be tempted to get all of the information you can. With the vast pool of knowledge on the internet, there is a multitude of information concerning the stages of pregnancy. However, you need to be careful because there are also people out there who put up information online that are not from trusted sources. Such information may convince you that you have symptoms of a pregnancy defect that you don't actually have. So be careful to get information from only reliable sources. Seek professional help when you are not sure about something.

Adjustment to changes

There will definitely be physical changes that accompany the state of pregnancy but there are many other changes you will also experience. For example, you will have to adjust to new responsibilities, including spending more money and having new work arrangements that will suit your new state. You will also have to adjust to changes in the form of your diet. Your doctor will guide you about the food that is not good for you and what will be helpful for your condition during this period. You will also have to adjust to being less active than before.

Gain weight

As much as you will be given a strict diet regimen as an expectant mother, you will gain weight. Exercise as much as you can and diet as you can, but you are most likely going to gain weight. There are rare cases of women who don't gain weight when they are pregnant. Such women often look as though they only have a basketball tucked under their dress. However, this is more of an exception rather than the rule. Therefore, don't be surprised to find out that you are gaining weight in unusual places—like your feet—as a mama-to-be.

Morning sickness

As a first-time mother, this might be new to you, but it is nothing new. Your body will change rapidly during pregnancy and it is likely you may develop nausea and throw up a few times. If this happens to you, don't be afraid. There is nothing wrong with you; it's part of the whole process. It is important that your doctor is your confidant during this period. It is safe to report anything you feel is unusual to your doctor. This will enable you to know when to act and when to be patient.

Physical changes in your body

Physical changes are also part and parcel of the changes you can expect when expecting. It is normal that your breasts become bigger and of course, your belly. Your body is simply getting set to nurture and deliver a baby. You will feel like eating more during this time and that is why you need to be careful about what you eat. Your hunger should not make you eat whatever comes your way. You should plan your meals and decide what should be part of your diet and what should not be. You really need the support of your family and friends during this period.

Taking leave from work

If you are a career woman, you should also expect to be granted leave from your work when you are expecting a baby. Only a totally unreasonable boss will not sanction leave for you, especially when your due date gets closer. A leave is your right as an expectant mother. This will allow you time to rest and take good care of yourself as you wait for the delivery of your child. You need to take advantage of your time off and put everything that is needed for your safe delivery in place.

Preparation for becoming a parent

It is obvious that by the time you deliver your beautiful baby, your status will change. You will become a mother— a parent. You will have to prepare for this upcoming situation by acquiring things like baby clothes. You should also expect that your friends who have been parents before you, as well as members of your family and your parents (if you still have them), will give you tips that can help you. Receiving the right information is vital when preparing for parenthood because it will help you excel as a parent.

New relationships

There are new beneficial relationships that will be formed during this time. It is a common practice to identify people that can help you and people who are similar to you. If you are the kind of person that has never had a cordial relationship with a medical practitioner before now, you will have a number of them as an expectant mother. Your doctor will be your good friend as well as other medical professionals you will need to consult at the hospital. Other pregnant women who come around the hospital will also offer you valuable support.

Cultural support

You will need all the help you can get as a pregnant woman, especially the support of people who share your cultural background. It is true that the world is a global village, today thanks to advancements in technology. And with modern medical facilities, giving birth to a child has never been easier. However, the emotional support of people who share cultural values will come in handy, especially during labor.

Irrational fear

No mother wants to lose her baby and I am sure you are no different. Therefore, there is the likelihood that you are being very careful about what to do and what not to do during this period so that you don't hurt yourself or your baby. Being careful is good; but problems arise when your caution grows into worry and eventually fear. Some people will tell you outrageous things, such as that being in a room where there is a running microwave will make your baby autistic. (This is not true; autism is genetic.) Therefore, it is always good that you get information from verified sources to avoid becoming unnecessarily fearful.

WHAT FATHERS SHOULD EXPECT WHEN THEY ARE EXPECTING

Expectant fathers have a mixed bag of reactions when their wives become pregnant. They are glad to know that Junior is on the way. However, they are also aware that there are adjustments and sacrifices that the journey to parenthood demands. Some of the most important things expecting dads have to look out for as they await the birth of their child are discussed below:

Quality support for the wife

No one should teach an expectant father that he has no part in offering quality support to his wife as she carries their baby. It is gross irresponsibility for a man to not realize that he needs to be committed to helping his wife deliver their baby successfully. The father needs to provide emotional support, financial support, and physical support for his wife in this period in particular. Failure to provide the requisite support will only stress the woman and make her burden more difficult to bear.

Less sex

Some people still assume that sex should not be mentioned in the same breath as an expectant woman. Interestingly, there are still people who believe that they will be hurting their soon-to-be-born baby if they have sex with their wife during pregnancy. This belief has no foundation. What is true is that the rate and intensity of sex will reduce but it is not true that sex is not safe for a pregnant woman. An expectant father needs to understand that the body of his wife is using up a lot of energy to develop the child and must be understanding with her when she complains of fatigue. The second trimester is the best phase of pregnancy for sexual activities because the woman will have more energy by then.

A fatigued wife

Fatigue is almost synonymous with pregnancy, because developing another human being demands a lot of energy from your body. It should not be a surprise that the woman complains of being extremely tired, especially during the first trimester. There is a lot of progesterone that is being supplied into the blood of the woman during this period and the result of this is that the woman will not be as active as she used to be and will feel like sleeping. She will most likely also go to bed earlier than she used to. An expectant father must be willing to understand and encourage her to see the doctor if she is complaining of being overly tired.

Pregnancy mood swings

A woman's emotions can be amplified by the reactions and changes in her body when pregnant. Therefore, veteran fathers understand that they need to be more patient and understanding with their wives when they are expecting a child. She can be moody and not interested in anything the man does to excite her or make her smile for a considerable part of the day. The last thing she needs from her man is him being angry or fussy. If things are not getting done around the house, bear with it and help out. She will return to her normal activities when she feels better.

More expenses

One of the most important forms of support an expectant father needs to provide for her wife while she is carrying their baby is financial support. The father-to-be must understand that the woman and their baby will need a lot of attention during this phase. It often demands a significant commitment financially. Therefore, an expecting father must start setting aside more money for the important things that need to be bought to alleviate her discomfort and help her through this challenging time.

Changes in daily routine

Pregnancy is a positive disruption of the daily routine of the home. The protruding belly of the woman will not only affect her body but will also sap her energy. The implication of this depletion of energy is that the woman will find it more difficult to carry out some of the activities the man has come to trust her to carry out in the home. This change will demand that the father be ready to take more responsibilities at this time. An expecting father must anticipate this change and be ready to adapt to it. A man's commitment and love will be tested during this phase of marriage.

Rearrangement of the home

As the couple prepares to welcome their baby, they will also need to make some changes in the home. They will need to acquire things like a stroller, nursing rocker, or a swing, and space will have to be found to accommodate these things. You will also want to purchase toys and other interesting gadgets, as long as they are safe for the baby. Some small rearrangements—or in some cases, major ones—will be needed. You may also want to decorate a nursery to welcome your new family member.

Stop smoking

The instruction to stop smoking is not relegated to just the pregnant woman, but also to the expecting father. Everyone in the household should avoid smoking, espccially inside, as you await the birth of the baby. Smoke, first- or second-hand, is not good for either the baby or the mother. A little caution can annul a major disaster.

Prenatal visits

Prenatal visits used to be seen as a woman's business, but that is no longer the case. The modern expectant father knows that he needs to accompany his wife for her prenatal visits. Of course, this does not mean that the father to be must be available for every visit, but it should be as much as possible. This is a further show of commitment and sacrifice which will mean a lot to the wife. Women are tempted to assume that the man is not as enthusiastic and committed to the birth of the child if he ignores this step. A simple way to counter that misconception is going with her for prenatal visits.

Learn more about the birthing process

The last phase of pregnancy is the very vital topic of the labor and birth of the child. The mother-to-be will learning all she can to ensure a successful delivery. The father-to-be is also expected to play a vital part in this. He can take birthing classes with her so that he can also learn as much as he can. This learning process will help him understand what is happening and how he can be of help to her as she labors. Pregnancy is a period that has the potential to make the bond between a husband and a wife stronger. The father is expected to contribute his efforts faithfully to take advantage of this opportunity.

NUTRITION BEFORE AND DURING PREGNANCY

What to take and what not to take before and during pregnancy is very important. Diet can affect your chances of getting pregnant. Your nutrition during pregnancy is critical to how easy or difficult the labor process will be for you. Your nutrition while carrying a child can also affect the health of your unborn child.

What to eat before pregnancy

You need to prepare your body before getting pregnant. Below are some important tips regarding your nutrition that will aid your bid to get pregnant:

Stronger bones with calcium

You need to develop stronger and healthier bones as you prepare your body for pregnancy. There is no better way to do this than to eat foods that contain calcium daily. Excellent sources of calcium include sardines, almonds, collards, bread, yogurt, cheese, beans, and lentils. When you finally get pregnant, this calcium will also make the child healthy. It is recommended that a woman who plans to get pregnant should have a daily intake of one thousand milligrams. Failure to do this puts you at risk of osteoporosis, a medical condition in which your bones are weak and can break easily.

More Iron

The natural monthly outflow of blood from your body during menstruation leaves your body deficient of the necessary amount of iron that you will need to carry a baby. Hence, it is important that you make up for this loss through the regular intake of iron. Good sources of iron include meat such as liver, pork, lamb, or beef. You can also get a substantial amount of iron from leafy greens like collards, kale, broccoli, and turnip greens, as well as whole grain bread and dry beans. Iron will not only help your body prepare to receive a child, but it will also improve the health of your child.

Take more folic acid

Your daily meal is not complete without 400mg of folic acid. This is the recommendation of U.S Public Health Service. Folic acid is important for the avoidance of birth defects that affect the spinal cord and the brain. An example of these defects is spina bifida, which affects the vertebrae such that they will not fuse together the proper way. The implication of this is that the spinal cord will be left exposed, which is very dangerous. Such exposure can lead to paralysis and even inhibited brain function. You can get folic acid from citrus fruits, nuts, green leafy vegetables, and cereals. Include these foods regularly in your meal to guarantee a healthy body that is set to nurture a well-developed baby.

What to eat during pregnancy?

It is important to note that calcium, iron, and folic acid are not only important for you before you get pregnant. You need them even more when you are pregnant. Apart from these aforementioned three, there are also other important nutrients your body needs during pregnancy. Some are listed here:

Go for more fruits and vegetables

The rich nutrients present in fruits and vegetables makes them important components of your daily meal. However, they become a paramount part of your daily food when you are pregnant. Fruits and vegetables are excellent sources of calories. You need more calories during pregnancy so as to be able to maintain your energy level. It is recommended that you increase your calories by 300, especially for the second and third trimester. What this means is that if you needed 2500 calories daily before you became pregnant, you will have to increase it to 2800 calories when you are carrying a child.

Include more proteins in your meal

Protein is another important nutrient that should not be missing from your daily diet. Your baby needs it for the building of body cells. There are a lot of changes that are taking place in your body when you are pregnant and you will need a substantial amount of protein to keep these processes going. For example, your body needs to build the placenta, which demands a lot of protein. As a pregnant woman, you will need 70g protein daily, which is 10g more than your daily requirement before pregnancy. Great sources of protein are milk, meat, fish, eggs, and tuna.

More fluid

Your body will demand more fluid when you are pregnant. You will find yourself being more thirsty than usual. Ensure you maintain a regular intake of water. Dehydration is the last thing you want to encounter as a pregnant woman. Eight to twelve cups of water should be your minimum daily amount. The nourishment that goes through the placenta from you to your baby requires a good supply of water for ease of passage.

Risky nutritional practices before and during pregnancy

There are some risky nutritional practices that you should not practice before or after pregnancy. They include:

- **Eating raw food-** Raw food or poorly-cooked food has the possibility of containing dangerous parasites that can hurt you as well as your unborn child. Tasty foods like sushi, poached eggs, raw seafood, and poorly cooked meat are susceptible to carrying bacteria that are dangerous to your health. Don't sacrifice your health or the health of your baby for the sake of taste.

- **Skipping meals-** People have various excuses for skipping meals, such as work schedules or loss of appetite. You will be hurting your body when you skip meals, especially when you either want to get pregnant or you are heavy with a child. In case you have issues with your appetite, you can talk to your doctor rather than let this poor nutritional practice linger. You need over 85,000 calories during the nine months of your pregnancy. The last thing you should do is miss any meals.

HOW A CHILD'S BRAIN WORKS: BASIC RULES AND THEORIES

It is important you understand how the brain of a child works as a parent to be because this understanding will help you train your child effectively when you eventually have one. The brain is the most important organ because it coordinates the other parts of the body. Therefore, an effectively working brain is vital for a fully functional individual. The brain is like a company that has various parts that work together that achieve a common goal.

Little geniuses

When you look at a child sometimes, you will have to marvel. They are little geniuses of communication, listening and imitation. The brain is the machine that coordinates all of these activities that looks simple on the surface but actually involves a whole lot of background activities that are complex but interesting to understand.

There are five parts of the brain, which all have different functions that are important to the daily activities of a child. They consist of the cerebrum, brain stem, cerebellum, hypothalamus, and the pituitary gland. Each one of them is discussed below:

Cerebrum

The cerebrum is the largest part of the brain. It is responsible for critical thinking and is also in charge of the voluntary muscles on the body. In other words, the child is able to move because of the activities that go on in the cerebrum. What that means is that when you see your child throwing a ball or waving his or her hand, the cerebrum is responsible for these. This part of the brain is also responsible for solving problems and playing games.

It is the site of both short-term and long-term memory as well. The cerebrum is divided into two halves on the right and left side of the brain. Neuroscientists believe that the right side is what helps the child understand things that cannot be seen or touched, like music. The left side is believed to be responsible for speech and logic. Interestingly, the right half of the cerebrum controls the left part of the body and vice versa.

The cerebellum

The cerebellum does not match the cerebrum when it comes to size but it is also responsible for important activities the child does. The cerebellum, which is found below the cerebrum, controls coordination, movement, and balance. It is the cerebellum that helps your child stand upright and maintain balance.

Brain Stem

The brain stem, like the cerebellum, is not large in size but has important functions all the same. It is responsible for the connection between the brain and the spinal cord. Every activity that has to do with being alive is in the care of this powerful part of the brain. Your child's breathing, circulation, and digestion are all thanks to the brain stem. The brain stem is also responsible for the activities of the involuntary muscles like blinking and pumping blood from the heart to the rest of the body.

Pituitary gland

Your child is only able to grow because of the pituitary gland. This organ, which is just about the size of a pea, creates and sends hormones into the body. As you marvel at the growth of your child, remember that it is because the pituitary gland is working properly. It is also responsible for the regulation of the amount of water and sugar in the body.

Hypothalamus

The easy way to understand this part of the brain is to think of a thermostat. The hypothalamus regulates the temperature of the body to ensure that it is neither too hot nor too cold. Interestingly, when you find your child sweating or shivering, it is the hypothalamus trying to bring the body back to an acceptable temperature.

Development of the brain during pregnancy

The neural plate is what can be described as a brain in a fetus. It eventually becomes the neural tube, which forms into four distinct parts called the forebrain, hindbrain, midbrain, and the spinal cord. All of this is completed within the first seven weeks of pregnancy. By the sixth week, your child is already able to carry out activities such as sucking, stretching, swallowing, and of course, breathing.

The part of the brain that develops last is the cerebral cortex. It is in charge of the voluntary actions of your child and will not be developed fully until some years after birth.

How to develop the brain of your child

There are things you can do that will help the brain of your child develop properly. They are discussed below:

Healthy food

The brain of your child requires minerals and vitamins that will help it grow and develop properly. You have an important role to play in this by ensuring that your child has a good supply of food that contains vitamins and minerals.

Proper hygiene

Good hygienic practices might not necessarily directly help the brain of your child develop but it will help you ensure that you don't interfere with the development of your child. Simple hygienic practices like washing fruits properly before eating, as well as wearing bug spray when you need to travel during the summer, will go a long way in helping your child avoid any major setback. Wearing bug spray is a precaution against the Zika virus, which can cause a major setback in the development of your child's brain.

Helpful activities

You can also help develop the brain of your child by letting the child do activities that involve distinguishing objects and exposure to pictures. Such activities will train the brain of the child to solve problems at an early age.

HOW WE UNDERSTAND OUR CHILD

Having a good understanding of your child, especially in the first few months after birth, is vital. It can create a platform for a solid rapport that will continue into adulthood. Your baby cannot express him or herself with words in the early months of life. This seeming lack of communication can be difficult to understand and frustrating, especially for new parents, who feel helpless to meet the needs of an ever-demanding child.

Interestingly, your child actually communicates in ways that will require you to pay proper attention to understand him or her. Below are some tips that can help you understand your child so that you can be the happy parent of a happy child:

The pattern of crying

For some people, all they can see when a child cries is a yelling and unhappy little one. However, the cries of a child are not for the sake of causing nuisance. It is an expression of a need to be met. If you are watchful enough, you will find out that the cries of your child take different patterns. A child who simply wants your attention when left to him or herself for a while might cry for five or six seconds and stop.

This stop is temporary, because the child is only waiting for the outcome. Failure will lead to another series of the same cry till the need is met. When your child is hungry, the cry will be the same as the first but louder when the child is not fed. The child can be more dramatic and be found moving his or her head around to tell you that the need is urgent.

Time to sleep

Babies sleep quite frequently, especially in the first few months. You can know when your child is telling you that it is time to sleep. He may become passive and seem to lack interest in playing with you. Don't stimulate the baby to play again when you notice this, because your effort may be futile and you will end up being disappointed.

Playtime

The interesting part of your child's playtime is that it is not in your control but dependent on the willingness of the child. Your baby will let you know when he or she wants to play and when he or she is no longer interested. When your child is ready to play with you, she will appear calm, with eyes that are wide open. It is likely that she will fix her gaze on your face. Your face is the most interesting play tool for your child in the early months. He will most likely replicate your gestures, like sticking out your tongue.

Rotating the head

Your baby can rotate his head to let you know that he is feeling like sleeping. This might also be a sign that your child is not comfortable being around people she is not used to. Rotating the head is also an indicator that your child is anxious and trying to calm down.

Lifting the leg

Unlike adults, babies are not able to adjust to pains. They can only attempt to let their caregivers know how they are feeling. Apart from crying, an important way your child can alert you to the fact that he is feeling pain is by lifting his leg.

Feeling uncomfortable

You can also know when your baby is feeling uncomfortable. This discomfort may be as a result of a soiled diaper. You may not really see this as a serious issue, but some babies frown at that. They will make their intention known by a show of restlessness or crying intermittently. By the time you change the diaper, you will realize what had been the issue. You can also detect this discomfort when your baby is not interested in playing.

Erratic movements

Your child might also be trying to pass a message across to you when you notice that she moves in an unusual way, like grabbing her ears. This can be meaningless, but you need to pay attention when you observe that your baby often does this and cries afterwards. It may be as a function of an infection that is not obvious to you. When that happens, don't hesitate to see your doctor as soon as possible. It is better for your doctor to confirm that there is no cause for alarm than for you to assume that all is well when it is not.

Clenching the fist

It is not too uncommon to see your baby clench his fist. This is often an indication of hunger. When you see your baby clenching his fist, it is a pointer to a rumbling stomach. When you don't give him the food he craves on time, he will move from clenched fists to crying. Taking timely action when you see your baby clench his fist will avert a bout of unpleasant crying that will follow soon.

Arching the back

Babies are fond of arching their backs for different reasons. When they are already full when you are done feeding them, they can arch their backs to let you know that they don't want any more food. Your baby might be having reflux if you notice that she regularly arches her back while she is eating. It is, however, important to note that these interpretations will only be applicable if your baby is two months old or less. If your baby is older, arching the back can be a sign of hunger or fatigue.

HOW OUR CHILD UNDERSTANDS US

It is not only parents that are saddled with the responsibility of understanding the child, but the child also has to understand the parents. Your baby is not only an active communicator; he or she is also an active listener. Their response is not often very fast but you can be assured that they can also listen to you and understand you.

You will be excited to hear your baby call you Mama for the first time, but your baby has been learning and understanding his environment long before then. You might be surprised to find out that your child learns actively. You might not notice the process but you will definitely see the results when they start manifesting. You also have an active role to play in helping your child understand you and his environment.

Early bloomers

It is amazing to know that your child begins to learn to respond and recognize signs and languages as early as a month old. Where the issue often lies is being able to distinguish between mere sounds and specific languages. This often takes them a while before they eventually catch on. So while you keep calling your baby by name, you are not speaking to the air; your child is gradually learning to know that she has a name that is distinct from the name of the objects and other people around her.

Receptive language

By the time your baby is five to six months old, he will be able to distinguish the meaning of peculiar sounds from the cacophony of sounds in the environment. This capacity to identify the meaning of sounds is the phenomenon called receptive language. Interestingly, your child will start being able to recognize your voice by the time she is three months old. She will be able to react to changes in the loudness of music as well as your change of tone between three months and six months. Between six months and a year old, she will be able to speak simple words like cup and bottle.

Latter phase

By the time your child is a year and a half, he will be able to understand combinations of words and respond accordingly. You will be able to tell him to carry out two separate activities that are unrelated or related like picking up a toy and putting it on the table. Your child's cognitive ability will further develop when he is almost two years old. He will be able to play with puzzles and solve easy ones by this stage. You can also start giving some toilet training to your child at this stage. The key part of toilet training is helping your child to see a connecting between easing himself and the potty.

How to help your child understand you faster

You have a vital role to play in ensuring that your child understands you and his or her environment faster. Below are some vital contributions that can help the understanding of your child:

Talk to your child regularly

Most parents talk to their babies before they are even born. However, it should not be an activity carried out because of the excitement of expecting a child. It should continue after the birth of the child because it is beneficial. The more you talk to your child, the more you will be able to help him or her have a good grasp of the difference between your voice and that of others. You don't have to just talk for the sake of it; you can read a storybook to your child in the early months. Your child will become very familiar with your voice this way. Apart from reading, you can also sing for your baby. You will help your child build a trusting relationship with you.

Introduce toys

You need to help your child understand space, orientation, and other important things in her environment. Toys that are proper for the age of your child will also come in handy. These toys will help her develop physically and mentally. She will be able to distinguish between various textures and shapes as she plays. She may have a favorite toy, having learned over time that toys are not the same. She will also learn that colors are not the same via this exposure to toys.

Don't be scared to say a lot

Some parents are careful of overwhelming their children and will not speak to them regularly because of that. As your child is still growing and developing, talking to him regularly will only help him develop his cognitive skills. Don't be afraid of overwhelming your child. He will let you know when he cannot take any more by becoming passive and disinterested when he is no longer interested in listening to you. So take advantage of every opportunity to help your child learn.

Get concerned in the event of passivity

Don't be excited about having a baby that is passive. It does not necessarily mean that your child has a calm personality. It might be that your child has issues that need to be resolved quickly. You really need to be concerned when your child is already two years old or more and does not have the capacity to respond to simple instructions. You should also be concerned if your child is not able to use a brush or a spoon. Talk to your doctor immediately so that you can find out if it is something you need to be patient about or treat as soon as possible.

YOUR PAST AFFECTS YOUR BABY

For every action, there is a reaction, says Sir Isaac Newton in his Third Law of Motion. This statement is not relegated to motion alone; it is a principle that is often at work in life. You have heard people tell you to focus on the future, especially when you have a rough past. It is indisputable that this advice is good but it does not change the fact that the past has a role to play in your future.

Your past affects you and your baby in two ways, either positively or negatively. The unique ways your past can affect your baby are highlighted below:

Abortion and premature birth

There are more myths than facts surrounding the issue of abortion. Some people assume that having an abortion will prevent you from having a normal pregnancy. Some people also think it makes you stand a higher risk of a miscarriage or low placenta. These claims are not accurate. However, an abortion increases your chances of premature birth. In the even that your womb gets infected after the abortion, your ovaries and fallopian tubes can also be affected. This infection, which is known as a pelvic inflammatory disease (PID), can lead to premature birth. The risk of being infected with PID can be reduced when you are given antibiotics prior to an abortion.

Obesity and asthma

It is often recommended that you shed excess weight before pregnancy because being fit will help you successfully overcome the rigors of labor. Moreover, another advantage of taking off excess weight is to avoid maternal obesity. Maternal obesity has been linked to an increase in the risk of a child being asthmatic. Hence, regular exercise is recommended for you before getting pregnant so that your baby is not affected by your past actions or inactions. If you are already pregnant, it is not too late. You can still take a long walk at least once a week, particularly in the first trimester.

Moderate caffeine

The appropriate level of caffeine for a pregnant woman has been up for debate for a while because, while some research suggests that excess caffeine will hurt your child, there is also research that posits that low levels of caffeine will affect the weight of your child. According to the American College of Obstetricians and Gynecologists, it is recommended that a pregnant woman should limit caffeine intake to 200mg per day, the equivalent of two cups of full-strength coffee. You need to be careful with the quantity of coffee you drink daily, because this can affect your baby.

Careless use of antidepressants

The frequent mood swings associated with pregnancy makes it tempting for women to take antidepressants when they are pregnant. However, you need to be careful about this because it can affect the development of your child. Birth defects and miscarriages have been linked to the use of antidepressants. Talk to your doctor about alternative treatment. Cognitive behavioral therapy, for example, is an effective therapy that can help you handle depression when carrying a child. You can contact a certified psychologist for more information. This does not involve medication, which makes it safer than the use of antidepressants.

Pay attention to your level of vitamin D

Low level of vitamin D has been linked to various health challenges for a baby such as low birth weight and gestational diabetes. Vitamin D is readily available, as it is the vitamin you get from sunlight. However, with the increasingly sedentary lifestyle of today's modern world, it is possible not to get enough. A lot of people today live in airconditioned houses, get into their cars and stay in airconditioned offices and return home. If you have this type of lifestyle, you need to do a test to check your level of Vitamin D before getting pregnant because this oversight can affect your baby.

Uncontrolled appetite and listeria

Listeria is not common among pregnant women but it can be devastating if a pregnant woman contracts it. Hence, it is better to be safe than sorry. Such women have a high chance of stillbirths, infection of the baby, and premature ejection. You can be infected by listeria when you have a poor habit of not washing fruits properly before eating them. You can also be affected by this disease when you eat processed meats like smoked salmon, deli meats, and hot dogs. You will feel like eating a lot when you are pregnant but you need to be careful so that your actions do not jeopardize the health of your baby.

Air pollution and low birth weight

Smoking cigarettes is dangerous, but that is not the only airborne toxin you may be exposing your unborn child to. There are air pollutants all around you, especially if you live in a city. You don't have to move just because you are pregnant, but you need to be careful to avoid air pollutants. Air pollution has been linked to low birth weight. Therefore, you will have to take extra care to avoid rush hour traffic and other sources of air pollution to safeguard the health of your unborn baby.

Your upbringing and child training

The demons of your home training can also rear their ugly heads, especially if you had parents who didn't treat you well. Most people who had unpleasant childhoods vow to ensure that their children do not experience the kind of treatment meted out to them. Interestingly, most parents who treat their kids badly were also treated that way by their parents. You will need to be deliberate in the way you train your child so that you don't repeat the mistakes your parents made.

WHAT IF I AM DOING IT WRONG?

Every good parent wants to give their children the best possible platform to excel in life. This uncharted new course makes parents-to-be a little nervous. You are not alone if you are anxious about parenting. You are being careful about making grave mistakes that can jeopardize the future of your kids. Rest assured that no one gets it right all the time. Below are helpful parenting tips for your perusal:

There is no parenting style that is the best

You will be starting on the wrong note if you already have a particular parenting style with which you want to train your child. I am not saying it is wrong to have standards that you want your children to follow; what I am saying is that you will have to be flexible with the way you train your kids. Some kids do better when you allow them to have their way a little and help them grow while some need you to be stern all the way.

You will not be helping your children if you have planned to train them with the same techniques your parents used to train you because it might not be applicable to them. Being flexible enough to develop a training pattern that best suits your kids is fundamental in raising children you will be proud to have.

You will make mistakes

You probably don't want to hear this, but you have to learn to accept that you will make mistakes in life generally, and being a parent is no different. You will make decisions you will wish in hindsight that you hadn't. The only solace you have is that you can choose to either reduce the rate at which you make mistakes or not. Being open to seeking knowledge from credible sources will help you to reduce the chances of making mistakes. No parents are perfect. The best parents are the ones who have learned to reduce their mistakes so that they don't hurt their children beyond measure.

Be a fast learner

You must be ready to learn the lessons that your mistakes as a parent teach you. The truth is that parenting is something you have to learn and will learn on the job. Great parents use their previous errors to make better decisions in the future. It is not bad to make mistakes as a parent because every parent makes mistakes at one point or the other.

However, it is very bad when you do not use your mistakes as a teaching tool. Anyone who does not have the capacity to learn from past mistakes is not an intelligent person. Veteran parents are products of experience, knowledge, and valuable lessons learned as a result of the wrong choices they made in the past.

Learn to forgive yourself

A key virtue you must have as a parent is the ability to move on quickly. There is a tendency to keep reminding yourself of the mistakes you have made in the past. It becomes more difficult to move on when the mistakes you made hurt your kids significantly. No good parent wants to hurt their children. Yet all parents hurt their kids once in a while. You have to forgive yourself and move on.

Feeling bad about your previous mistakes for too long will only make you too emotional to make the right decisions in the future. You will only set yourself up for further mistakes when you are clouded by how you feel. You will deprive yourself of the requisite capacity to make logical decisions, which will only hurt you and your kids further. You need to let go because you still have the chances to right your wrongs if only you will learn to forgive yourself and always be ready to start again. Better days are ahead if only you take your eyes off the bad days of the past.

Apologize if you are wrong

Some parents are so proud that they feel it is inappropriate to apologize to their kids when they have hurt them. The mindset that parents don't have to apologize to their children is archaic and should not be encouraged in the modern world. Your kids will learn to forgive you when you have wronged them but you will make the process of their healing faster when you are humble enough to let them know that you are sorry about what you did to them.

Your decision to apologize to your kids is never wrong. It will only make the bond between you stronger. Your kids might assume that you don't care about them and hurt them intentionally when you refuse to apologize for your actions. Apologies make your intention clear to your kids. Your children will know that you are not perfect and will accept and love you all the same as they grow older. You will make the journey easier for both you and them when you are quick to let them know that you did not hurt them intentionally.

Walk your talk

Setting a good example is a key ingredient in parenting. You confuse your children when your actions do not match your words. Whatever character you want to instill in your children must be demonstrated by you. Children learn more by observing you than the words you speak. They will remember the things you do more than the things you say. You are the first teacher your kids have and they will assume that you are always right till they have further exposures in life. You cannot afford to lose the respect of your children because of your inconsistencies. Always set a good example for them to follow.

EVERY CHILD IS DIFFERENT

You will not be doing your kids any favor when you treat them as the same. Things get worse when you compare your kids with other people's and you expect them to adhere to the same standards. Successful parenting does not follow the same procedure. There is nothing set in stone when it comes to parenting. You will only make your home consistently tense when you assume that all kids are the same and should be made to go through the same routine. Kids are different in the following ways:

Rate of learning

One of the worst myths in the world is that all kids learn at the same rate. This is often evident in school. Some kids are able to carry out the things they have been taught almost immediately, while some take a longer time to learn. They will get it eventually, but you will need to be patient. The great Albert Einstein was seen as a dysfunctional child when he was younger but he eventually overcame his learning difficulty. Do you want to raise an Einstein? Then you will need to be patient with your kids when they seem to be learning at a slow pace.

Personalities

The personality of your kid is like a flower that blooms slowly. You will begin to see it gradually unravel as they grow older. Kids have different personalities. One child may be very active and talk constantly, while the next has a calm, quiet demeanor. Don't be too pushy or make your kids feel bad because they are not exhibiting the same characteristics you notice in other kids. Your children are unique and the best you can do for them is to love them for who they are. Comparison with other kids will only break his spirit and make him withdrawn, believing you don't appreciate him.

Challenges

You cannot expect a child who has a genetic issue or injury in the early years to be able to compete favorably with kids who do not have the same challenge. You have an important role to play to ensure that your kids do not give up on themselves because of their challenges. There are many examples of people who had learning difficulties and other issues who later achieved great things. In case you have a child in this category, don't wish you have another. Treat the child well. Your support and love is a vital ingredient that will help the child overcome her challenge.

Strengths

Children do not have the same strengths. There are some things that your child will do well that other kids will struggle to do. In the same way, there are some capabilities you will see some kids display you can only wish your kids would display too. Some kids excel in sport while others do better in activities that have to do with logical reasoning and analytical skills. Encourage your kids to build on their strengths and help them get better in areas where they are weak. Patiently help your kids grow and avoid the temptation to put unnecessary pressure on them.

Vulnerabilities

In the same way that kids don't have the same strengths, they also have different vulnerabilities. The best thing you can do for your child is to help him know that you love him in spite of his vulnerabilities. You will not be helping your kids when you constantly criticize them. Help them find ways to improve themselves, but you must let it be apparent to them that you are their biggest fan at different stages of their development. Don't blame yourself for their vulnerabilities because it does not necessarily mean you have done something wrong or are doing something wrong.

Social skills

Some kids have incredible social skills that endear them to many people within a short time. Such children make friends easily wherever they go. Others are not like that. They have rich inner worlds and are not quick to make friends. You can help your child develop better social skills, but you should not make your child feel unwanted because he or she is having difficulty relating to others. Your kids must see you as their best friend and this will eventually extend to the way they relate with other people. You should not mix up the personality of your kids with their social skills. Having poor interpersonal skills is not the same thing as being an introvert. The social skills of your kids are not set in stone; they can be improved.

Celebrate the uniqueness of your kids

The moment your kids are not sure whether you love them or not, you are already failing in your duties as a parent. It must be crystal clear to your kids that you appreciate them. Don't force her to become a doctor because it is your ambition for her when it is clear that she excels in art. When you jettison the unique abilities of your kids, you are already trying to make them who they are not. Once they lose their uniqueness, they have lost what makes them special.

Part Two

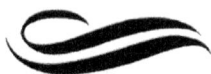

Myths and Legends

There are so many concepts in the world today that are not true. Some myths have stayed so long that people automatically assume they are true. The problem with myths is that they will mislead you and guide you into practices that will hurt you and your loved ones. Some of the myths around the world today were circulated by misinformed journalists who wrongly reported certain "advancements" in knowledge from new research. In this part, some myths about parenting and child development will be busted. Get set to learn some life-changing facts!

HOW A CHILD'S BRAIN DEVELOPS: MYTHS AND FACTS

It is often difficult to dissociate facts from myths regarding the way the brain of a child develops. Below are myths and the facts about how the brain of your child develops:

Myth #1: Inert brains

There is a misconception that the brains of children are initially inactive. The implication of this myth is that people assume that babies do not have the capacity to hear or see in the early days of their birth. Therefore, you might have heard someone caution a new mother about speaking to her newborn since the child cannot hear. However, this is a wrong knowledge because babies begin to learn even while they are still in the womb! The birth of your baby is a continuation and not an initiation of learning.

Contrary to popular belief, your baby can also see from birth. According to the American College of Obstetricians and Gynecologists, at the 26th week of pregnancy, your child's eyes are fully formed and can sense light and see images. There have been rumors circulating that babies are only able to see objects that are very close to them but that is not true. Your baby can see objects at any distance. The issue is that they don't have the ability to control the muscles of their eyes, which results in them not being able to focus on specific objects. This lack of proper focus is the reason why it often takes a lot to make your child focus on you or look at the camera when taking pictures.

Myth #2: Sophisticated toys aid intelligence

It is true that toys can keep your children occupied as they play with them around the house. However, you need to be careful not to overestimate the importance of toys. For example, your kids will not become smarter because they have toys. Babies learn by having a feel of their surroundings regularly. They learn to overcome various challenges that obstruct them and become smarter as a result.

A toy is part of the environment and will help them, but it is not about the toys but the exploration of the environment generally. Don't let anyone pressure you into buying sophisticated toys because the promise that they will make your kids smarter is not realistic. It is better to expose your child to a stimulating environment rather than to spend a considerable part of your budget on toys.

Myth #3: Only kids should play

Saying that play is only meant for kids only deprives the mother of having fun and the child from learning as much as possible. You will help your child learn faster when you are part of the play. Don't allow traditional beliefs to make you lose a vital opportunity to connect to your baby in a very simple but special way.

As you put your baby on a mat or blanket for a tummy time, join the fun! Sing for your cute one and stimulate her to the fullest. A busy schedule may prevent you from participating in this rite regularly but you must participate in your child's play as much as possible. Get down to his or her level and experience some nice Mommy and baby time!

Myth #4: The Mozart effect

Just as I have pointed out earlier concerning the misconceptions that were birthed by misguided journalists, the Mozart effect ranks high on the list of such misconceptions. It is believed that children do better in their studies after listening to Mozart. This myth can be traced to 1992 when it was reported that according to a research that was carried out at the University of California, the grades of students who listened to Mozart for twenty to thirty minutes was better than that of students who didn't.

Some other researches posited that a certain part of the brain is stimulated that makes people better in the performance of certain tasks. There has never been any proof that this same research is applicable to babies. However, just like much wrong stuff in the media today, a lot of people assume that their babies will become more intelligent when they listen to Mozart. It is important to note that the best music for your child is your own voice.

Myth #5: Brain development is genetic

Some parents assume that they have no control over the development of the brain of their kids because they have an assumption that brain development in children is genetic. The nature versus nurture debate will never end but the development of the brain of your child has a lot to do with the environment. You have an important role to play in how your baby's brain develops. Activities as simple as talking to your child and reading books to him will help your child develop more than you think.

Your interaction with your baby enhances the vocabulary of your child. New words are being added daily and you will find that the first few words your child speaks were the same words you spoke to him or her. Hence, when it comes to the development of the brain of your child, you will be wrong to take a backseat because that approach will not help your child.

Myth #6: Delay in speech is normal

Don't let anyone convince you that it is normal when your child has speech issues. Before your child is ten months old, he or she will most likely only blab. By ten months old, your child should be able to say dada and mama. By the time your child is a year old, he or she should be able to combine some syllables. If this is not the case, speak with your doctor, because your child could have developmental issues that require medical help.

Some developmental issues become permanent and affect the child all through her life when not resolved early enough. If you notice that your child is not developing a good grasp of language, see your doctor for a checkup so that you will be able to ascertain whether treatment is required or not. The assumption is equivalent to carelessness, which is not an attribute you should have as a parent.

HOW PARENTS INFLUENCE THEIR CHILD'S DEVELOPMENT: MYTHS AND FACTS

Without a doubt, parents have a vital role to play when it comes to the development of their children. However, some of the popular presupposed influences parents have on the development of their children are either overrated or underrated. In this part, we will look at the assumptions and what is really obtainable regarding the influence you can have on your child as a parent:

Myth #1: Respiratory allergies are transmitted from the parents to the children

People often posit that children of parents with respiratory allergies will also contract these same allergies. Contrary to popular opinion, it is not true that your kid will be affected by the respiratory allergens that affect you. I am not in any way claiming that heredity does not have a role to play in this regard because that would also be false. What I am saying is that the impact of heredity when it comes to respiratory allergies is minimal.

For example, a child can have allergies that the parents do not have. There are different things that can make a child allergic. Heredity is just one of them, and not the whole story. In case your child has respiratory allergies or any other form of allergy, it is better you speak to your pediatrician rather than assume that your child is a victim of destiny.

Myth #2: Too much attention is bad

In the bid to train responsible kids, some parents think they need to deprive their kids of some level of attention so that they will learn to handle themselves properly. Babies are often seen as the culprit in this situation. Some parents feel that babies only cry to get attention, which they see as being selfish. This is ridiculous!

There is no such thing as spoiling a baby. In the event that your baby is crying and you pick him up and he ceases to cry, the fact is that the baby actually needed to be picked up at that point in time. It is important that your baby has the assurance that you will be there for him, especially in the first six months of life. According to the author of "Emotionally Intelligent Parenting," Maurice Elias, your baby needs to be sure that he or she can trust you to respond during the time of need.

Myth #3: Psychiatric disorders are products of bad parenting

Some people try to put everything that goes wrong with a child at the doorstep of the parents. One of these ridiculous attempts is how some assume that it is bad parenting that causes psychiatric disorders. This claim is atrocious and false. It is true that the environment of the child, as well as the nature of the relationship between the parent and the child, can aggravate a psychiatric disorder.

However, it is not true that a child can have psychiatric disorders as a result of bad parenting. Don't let anyone scare you unnecessarily regarding the way you train your child. You have to do everything within your capacity to offer your kid the best parenting because so many things can go wrong that can affect the health and future of the child, but psychiatric disorders are not a product of poor parenting.

Myth #4: Holding a book too close to the face of your child will damage the child's vision

This is another popular conjecture that you have to discard. It is one of those half-truths that have existed for so long that you may find it difficult to believe that it is not true. If you need to put a book close to the face of your child before she can see the page can be a symptom of bad vision and not the cause of it. In other words, it can be an indicator that the child needs to be treated but it is never the reason your child's vision is impaired.

If your child always insists that you bring a book closer to him or her, it does not necessarily mean that the child has bad vision. It might simply be a matter of preference. Moreover, if you have any doubt, you can always speak to your pediatrician to confirm if it is an issue that has to be corrected or nothing to worry about. Such guidance from experts is always a safe option rather than so-called popular beliefs.

Myth #5: You can't raise healthy children if you are not wealthy

People speak the language of money these days and it has affected the value system of a lot of people. It is common to hear people make a statement like "If it is not making money, it is not making sense." As much as money is an important commodity in the modern world, its impact is often overrated. Don't let anyone bully you into thinking that your child will not turn out well if you are not wealthy.

It is true that there are things you will be able to afford when you are financially independent that will aid in the growth of your child, but there are cheaper alternatives that will not hurt him. Being wealthy does not automatically mean that a person will raise a healthy kid; in fact, it may lead to giving the child things that are not needed, which can end up having adverse effects on the child. Quality hygiene and proper diet is key to raising a healthy child and not just your spending power. A deep pocket will not buy you a healthy child. So get your priorities right and stop getting carried away by fantasies.

GOOD AND BAD BEHAVIOR MYTHS AND FACTS

Parents often engage in wishful thinking such as saying, "God will protect me because I am good." New parents tend to see themselves as invulnerable to bad outcomes and are also unaware of what behavior is acceptable. They can hold unhealthy myths about the growth of their children. We will now discuss some general misconceptions about the good and bad behavior of your child.

Myth #1: Bribing your child will result in good behavior

You will agree with me that reinforcement of your child's good behavior as he is growing up is good. Most parents have at some time had to persuade their kids with gifts in other for them to keep behaving well. The fact is that bribing your child for good behavior every time is absolutely wrong and bad. Although at the beginning of development, many of his actions will have to be consciously reinforced to encourage continuation, you have to carefully exercise control over this as he grows.

Yes, moral development depends on you, but you have to use your moral development skills wisely. This is because, when you excessively bribe your child to behave well, she will always respond to the bribe because it is what she intended to gain in the first place. She begins to relate to good behaviors as incentive motivated. You should also know that if you have to give your child a gift to do something good all the time, definitely, you are creating a neural network and association that she does not have to behave well except she is given something for it.

Myth #2: Punishment is the only way to stop bad behavior

The truth is that punishment is not the only way to stop bad behavior. While it may be effective e, it is not the best way to stop your child from acting badly. Punishment can take many forms such as spanking, withdrawing play times, and/or grounding your child. While spanking for some children after several times of warning may lead to the elimination of such bad behavior, it will not work for other children; it can even make them more resistant to change to your desired behavior. As the child begins to grow and explore the home, he will need reactions from you in order to differentiate his behaviors. It is important to note that spanking and other physical punishments are not acceptable forms of child training.

Also, as your child begins to differentiate good and bad with words, you should begin to shape her behavior by communicating with her. Your communication will eventually manifest into how well she will respond to changing the unwanted behavior. For example, you can sit her down and have a conversation on why her behavior is unacceptable. Rather than just punishing her for behaving badly, you can frown, showing your disappointment in the behavior and make your intention known about having a talk about it right there or later. This will teach the child respect, and help her want to listen to you. She will have confidence in asking you how she can behave better in order to not displease you in the future.

Myth #3: You spoil your child by picking him up when crying

This is often associated with behavior development of little kids. When a little child cries, it may be as a result of pain, or displeasure about not getting something he wants. In whichever way, his cry is to get attention from you. Every parent will want to satisfy their child with the emotional support he needs. Your baby's most basic need is trust and safety. When your child cries and you pick her up, and then she stops after having been picked up, this action of yours simply means you are telling her that you are reliable, and a trusted source of support.

This goes a long way into the development of your child into adolescence and adulthood. From infancy, your kid is in the process of finding out and exploring her world. Picking her up when she cries helps her to develop a good personality because of the attention you give her. Carrying her does not infer that she has been spoiled and does not correlate with good or bad behavior. Sometimes she just needs a hug or support when she cries.

Myth #4: Boys are more active than girls

For years, we have been taught the misconception that male children are more hyperactive than girls. Due to this myth, parents have held incorrect ideas about their children's behavior. Do not let this stereotype make you develop a negative opinion about your child. In fact, girls are predisposed to a kind of inattentive hyperactive activity, while male hyperactivity mostly can be destructive. Essentially, either a male or female child can develop ADHD, but it is mostly on a mild level.

Although there are likely to be some cases where a girl can be destructive in her activities, you should not conceive the notion that something is wrong, but rather caution and shape her in the right direction. The activities they choose to engage in can be good predictors of their interests. Either way, boy or girl, your child hyperactivity is not a correlate of gender.

Myth #5: Children always throw tantrums to get their way

This in a way is like myth #3. But you need to know that your child is just beginning his life. While developing, tantrums are just one of those normal behaviors he will definitely display. People who say children who throw tantrums are bad are from the school of thought that treats children as little adults. Such people assume that kids have every mental capacity to understand the world just like adults and should be expected to act like adults. This incorrect mindset that has led to some people making children carry out strenuous jobs that are meant for adults. Let your child be a child. Tantrums are just one of those things being a child is all about.

Don't be misled to think that your child does this as a result of bad behavior; all that is needed is your attention. When you see him display this behavior, take time with him because what he needs is you and you alone. Your child needs to be assured repeatedly that he has your back and you should not shudder in your responsibility to affirm your love for him at every opportunity. When you assume that tantrums mean that your child is misbehaving, you will be unduly harsh with your child and punish him unnecessarily out of sheer frustration.

Myth #6: Serving your kid after rejecting it will spoil your child

Society has taught that a parent has to be assertive with children because they may become excessively choosy. But the truth is that it is not so. For example, from a study of toddlers, it was discovered that toddlers may try a new kind of food about fifteen times before they get adjusted to it. As a matter of fact, when babies do not take a particular food, it is because they are trying to allow their taste buds to adapt to it. Rejection of food for babies is mostly an adjustment thing.

As your child grows, he may also reject food by choice. This is not a matter of good or bad behavior. Probably you are not diversified enough in your cooking or you are becoming routine in your food preparation. You can also imagine eating the same kind of meal over and over again every two to three days. This can overly become boring to you. You will want to try new dishes, right? Yes. Adjust and modify your cooking styles for her so as to prevent the rate of rejecting food.

Myth #7: You reinforce bad behavior when you comfort your child

Parents have believed that comforting your baby is some sort of reward or that you are encouraging bad behavior enhancer when you comfort him. When your child shows displeasure about something and you comfort him, you are teaching him that he cannot always have everything he desires. You are telling him to show contentment. Your child is still growing, and even when adults get disappointed, they often withdraw and feel emotionally down.

You show strength by comforting your child when she's lonely, maybe due to resistance from you simply withdrawing. Even after spanking or punishing your child, you should not leave her in isolation for long. Take full responsibility for monitoring her to see her behavior afterward. If withdrawal or isolation comes up, you should comfort her with a soothing voice, emphasizing your displeasure in her behavior. This is an ideal way of helping your child change from bad to good behavior.

PARENTAL CONTROL: MYTHS AND FACTS

You may be tempted by innovative ideas that can help guide your child. As reported, about 39% of parents reported using technological parental controls for filtering, selecting and regulating their activities. A parental control involves time, activities or content restrictions and then monitoring your child's safety.

Children are also human. They are not to be controlled. If you try excessively to control them, they will not respond well to you. Rather than trying to get control-based solutions to your concerns, you should put your energy into finding connection-based solutions and mechanisms. Controlling them may be successful for a short time, but connection will last forever.

Myth #1: Failure to respond to all bad behaviors with a firm hand will make you lose control of your child

This myth can pose a serious concern for modern parents. You can make yourself obsessive about dealing with every instance of unacceptable behavior. For instance, if you are on a visit to a friend and your child suddenly exhibits aggressive and destructive behavior, you do not have the time to react like you would on a normal day at home. You do not want to spoil the fun of a day out with your child, so responding to every bad behavior with a firm hand is not a practical goal to have.

The main thing to keep in mind is that you child should understand that, even if you do not discipline them on the spot, you are not going to let things go. They should not think that just because you are not reacting immediately they are going to get away with bad behavior.

Myth #2: Parents control their kids' fate

Some parents often think of themselves as having total responsibility for their children's fate. This idea poses a heavy and unrealistic emotional burden on parents and their kids. In line with this belief, when kids have a problem, they feel they are a failure and have disappointed their parents by not living up to their expectations. The fact is that you cannot determine how your child's life and personality will turn out. You have to get that idea out of your mind. At some point your child will assert their independence, thereby creating a niche for themselves by separating from you.

Also, certain elements both internal and external have a potential influence on your child. You will agree with that even within your family, there are striking individual differences. Intelligence, mood, personality and temperament are different for every person. Even though these variations exist, parents are still very much responsible for caring for everyone's needs and making them feel loved and internalizing societal rules into them. Yes, even though you do all these things your only responsibility is to influence and shape them, but you cannot control their lives.

Myth #3: Compulsive sharing increases good social skills and generosity

Of course, it is love that makes you share. You cannot force your kid to share with others. This is very common among parents. You need to understand that children have minds of their own and you cannot just impose your values on them. The fact is that forcing your child to give up his possessions is likely to mean that he will become less empathetic and less generous later in life. At most, you should ask the question, "Honey, why don't you want to share your toy?"

The response you get will then help you to know what is lacking and from there you can engage her on the need to share. Over time, your lovely kid will begin to want to try giving to others rather than clinging to her things. Another thing you need to know is that if you always force your child to share their things, you may be teaching her irresponsibility and unaccountability. When your child does things like sharing things of her own volition, she becomes responsible for the outcome, and that will continue into future behavior at adulthood.

Sharing also comes from liking. If your child does not like someone, there is no connection with them. Also, as your child develops into an adult, he will be to discern whom he wishes to relate with if you do not force him to share while younger. But if it is the other way, when you force your child into compulsive giving or sharing, you are teaching him that if you want something and the person you want it from does not give it to you, you can take it anyway since sharing is compulsory. This idea is so entrenched in our society today that parents feel it necessary to make their kids share things with the hope that it will promote social skills and make them good people.

Myth #4: Child self-control comes from you making rules for your child

Self-control comes from self-discipline and self-discipline is a product of recognizing the best behavior at any point in time. There is no need for self-control if you are being controlled by others. You can imagine living by the rules your grandparents passed on to your parents. How cumbersome it would be to live by them in this generation. This is different from the chores the child is expected to do every day such as washing the dishes, tidying their room, etc.

When you make rules for your kid, you have already set the limits to which they can go in life. You have automatically designed the manifestation of her thoughts. Even if your kid believes she can do anything, your rules will always bring down the thought to conform to your leadership. Another danger of this rule to your kid is that it creates a gap or bridge between your child and you. She will definitely be relating with you based on the rules you have laid down and I am sure you do not want to create distance between you because you think setting rules will make her learn self-control.

There are ways to encourage your child to develop self-control, such as: showing empathy, meeting his needs, modeling self-control, and finally, understanding his capabilities and not anticipating more than his brain development allows.

Myth #5: Routine is good for children

The beginning of boredom that will eventually gravitate to depression is a routine life. Nobody wants the same thing the same way every day. This myth is similar to #4 but different. If your child wants to make a routine plan for her daily activities, let it be done by her. Whatever she comes up with on the plan is her business, not yours. You should avoid setting up a strict schedule for your child as this is dangerous and may lead to an inhibitory psychological lifestyle.

Myth #6: Not quitting encourages commitment

This is not entirely true. There is always a saying the doing something the same way over and over again will not change the result. Only when you do it in different ways can you learn how to do it better. There is no point making your child fixated on something if he does not have interest in doing it. Many parents have fallen for this belief that not allowing children to quit activities such as a certain sport will encourage commitment. This is not so.

The fact is that when you allow your child to try many things, he will eventually find a particular interest which he will show dedication and commitment to. You should also know that you do not own your child's heart. He will only be where his mind is even though you are trying to force him to keep participating in an activity he is struggling with. Another reason he might be failing to do well in an activity may be because of his teammates. It takes understanding to inquire into this and teach your child to adapt and maintain a good relationship with them.

CHILDREN'S REFLEXES: MYTHS AND FACTS

If you do not learn to notice and pay attention to certain behaviors in your child, then you are likely to be surprised with what your child will turn out to be when he/she grows up. It is not suggested that you overlook your baby's reflexes as this is essential to your child development and you personally.

Myth #1: My child is lazy and does not want to walk around. He could have cerebral palsy.

It is true that children are innately inquisitive and eager to move around and explore their environment. One sign of mild to moderate cerebral palsy is a gross motor development delay. A child who has gross motor delays will find it difficult to achieve critical physical movement milestones like rolling, sitting and crawling. He may reach these milestones later than his peers, or maybe not at all. A child's lack of movement is important and you need to be concerned about this, especially if he was born prematurely and has other symptoms of cerebral palsy. He may have muscle stiffness which could keep him from moving at the appropriate time. Never assume anything; always speak to your pediatrician. Interestingly, you may be right. It is possible that you find out after meeting your doctor that your child is only being lazy and needs to be given the proper stimulation in the environment that will encourage him to start moving and displaying better mastery of motor skills. However, if you are wrong, you will be making a serious mistake that can affect the future of your child drastically. Hence, it is always safe to speak to your pediatrician before you make any conclusion.

Myth #2: Any child with cerebral palsy will not mature to become an independent adult

If you fail to take responsibility concerning your child's reflexes and movement, she may suffer from cerebral palsy, quadriplegia or spastic dystonia. Children with spastic diplegia and hemiplegia can become adults with jobs and even families. If your child has cerebral palsy, it is recommended that you encourage her to work toward self-care and make herself more mobile. It is not true that no child with cerebral palsy will be able to live an independent or satisfying life. No case of cerebral palsy is the same. Talk to your pediatrician for a diagnosis and advice on how to help your child. You should not take the health of your child lightly and that is why you need to involve your doctor in any issue no matter how insensitive you think it is. Some health concerns can be averted if you are proactive enough and consult your doctor from the onset.

Myth #3: My child has cerebral palsy, so he will need a special school.

This myth, like many similar ones, is absolutely false. Many children with this disease tend to have only physical disabilities like walking and running, not mental disabilities. The two most likely walking problems are poor balance and control. In this present age of advancement in neonatal care, your child's mental ability can be retained if he has cerebral palsy. Even though cerebral palsy affects many parts of a child's developmental functioning, his mental ability will be normal. Before jumping to conclusions about the effects cerebral palsy can have on your child, talk to your doctor. The danger of not talking to your doctor first is that you can either overrate or underrate the impact of the dysfunction on the day-to-day activities of your child and one of these two will be helpful for your child. If you overrate the impact of cerebral palsy on your child's activities, you will assume that some activities are impossible for him and that will deny your child the opportunity to further develop in some areas of his or her life. If you underrate the impact of cerebral palsy on your child, you will have false expectations because you will assume that he can carry out some activities that he may be unable to do. It is always best to ask your doctor specific questions regarding the activities in which your child can participate and the ones he does not have the capacity to.

Myth #4: Babies have quiet sleep patterns

Babies' sleep is not quiet. There are often sudden jerks or twitches of the arms or legs. This is normal at all ages, not just for babies. Don't begin to look for issues when there are none. It is normal that you are concerned about your child but you must always ensure that your care is not based on emotions but verifiable facts. In case you are not sure whether the sleeping pattern of your child is normal, seek professional advice. Your pediatrician is in the best position to educate you on what is a normal or abnormal sleeping pattern so that you know exactly when to be worried and when there is no cause for alarm.

Myth #5: Children who make certain breathing sounds and noises are abnormal

Throat noises are caused by the passing of air through normal saliva or refluxed milk. The gurgling noises may build up during sleep. So, little by little, babies will begin to swallow their saliva more often. Nose noises are usually because of dryness. When a baby's nostrils are blocked, her feeding will be affected. Even you as an adult cannot eat when your nose is blocked, right? So when your child shows discomfort during eating, you need to check to make sure that her nose is not blocked. Don't begin to think that you are an expert suddenly because you have been nursing your child for a while.

Pediatricians are not only trained, but they also have extensive experience in every health situation you may come across when nursing your child. Speaking to him or her will help you know whether the breathing sound your child makes is normal or not. It is too risky to assume anything when it comes to nursing a child. You need to make your pediatrician your friend. Don't hide anything regarding the health of your child from him so that he will know how best to help you. Never forget that the diagnosis of your pediatrician may not be accurate if you either provide false information or refuse to let her know about some of the things you notice about your child that are not clear to you.

There is nothing personal when it comes to health issues, so don't hide any information from your doctor. Doctors are not just trained to diagnose and treat ailments; part and parcel of their training is the responsibility to keep whatever you discuss with them private and confidential. If you notice that your doctor speaks to a third party about your professional dealings without your consent, you have every right to report them to the appropriate authorities. It is also in your best interest to ensure that you patronize medical experts who have the right pedigree and history of quality health delivery before you take your child to them. Health matters are too delicate for immature professionals that cannot be trusted.

Myth #6: Your baby sneezes so she has an allergy

Sneezing helps to open and clear the nose. It may be caused by dust, fuzz or any strong odors. When your baby keeps sneezing when eating, then check the environment where he/she is being fed. You may be wearing too much perfume, which could be causing irritation in your child's nasal cavity. If the sneezing becomes consistent, then get nasal washes.

A CHILD'S CRYING: MANIPULATION OR A SIGNAL? MYTHS AND FACTS

Modern parents have often reported that they feel helpless and frustrated when they are unable to console their crying child. You should know no child or even grown adult would want to start crying for no reason. You must also be aware that the day you decided to have a child, you agreed to be your child's number one comforter. So the responsibility lies on you.

Myth #1: Children who cry often are likely to have personality disorders when they grow up

This is wrong to assume. As I said earlier, no human wants to cry for no reason. There is no correlation between crying during childhood and adulthood. There are several reasons why your child could be crying, and this could be from distress, attention-seeking like clinging, or hunger. If you've just fed your child a few minutes before and now he is crying again, you should go ahead and give him more. It could be that his metabolism rate is fast. Feed your child until he is filled.

You may also apply some soothing on the back of your baby to make her stop crying and feel your presence. Try rubbing her back to help relax. However, if the child persists in crying, you should get in touch with your doctor. You may have to state the number of times in each day, how long she cries, and the intensity of the cries as well.

Myth #2: Baby crying even though they are fed is not normal

Crying serves an absolutely important function in babies and it is generally normal in children. When they cry, the vocal cords are exercised and they learn awareness of their mouth, the sounds produced, tongue, and lips. This purpose is seen as necessary for later developmental and communication skills. Can you imagine your baby not making any noise or crying since birth? You would be definitely be concerned. Crying is necessary and important.

Myth #3: Crying always means something is wrong

When a child cries, it is not necessarily that there is something specific wrong; he could just simply need help from you. For example, some babies have a routine of crying anytime they are about to sleep. What you need to do is to pat or tuck him to sleep. Some babies might even need you to sing for them to sleep or hold them in your arms and read books to them. Don't worry, your baby does not understand your song or the book you are reading, but your body contact and the sound of your voice is all that he needs to calm down and stop crying.

Myth #4 Crying babies is a sign of bad parenting

Actually, because of the frustration, many parents take their baby's cry personally, as if it is a sign of bad parenting. Even though parenting is a skill, no parent no matter how expert, will be able to soothe and console their kid every time she cries. If your baby still keeps crying after you have done every possible thing to calm her down, just relax yourself. Keep assuring yourself that she is not hungry, in pain, or wet. You should be reminded that it is normal for infants to be occasionally restless.

Myth #5: Allowing a child to cry is bad

If your child happens to be struggling with a toy, let him fumble. When this happens, he may get displeased and cry. When he wails a bit, a new skill will be learned. This is because when a child copes with minor frustrations, it serves as a learning opportunity. Another case is when your child cries because you are establishing a bedtime routine for him. You should enforce bedtime so that everyone in the house, including you, can have enough rest.

This does not mean that you should let your child cry to sleep. It is not the first option, but if you have tried every technique to get her to sleep and she still refuses to sleep but wants to cry, letting her cry might be the only choice. Medical practitioners have suggested that this is harder on parents than on the baby. Psychologically, this will teach the child that her parents will not always be there for her and maybe sometimes, she will not need them.

LIFE IS MUSIC: MYTHS AND FACTS

The idea of music and child development is one of the most pervasive myth parents have been taught. The correlation started with the Mozart effect in 1993 when researchers showed that college students who listened to a Mozart sonata did better on a complex reasoning test. After this time, it became a popular theory that the Mozart effect influenced intelligence in children. It even got to the extent that a onetime governor of Georgia, Zell Miller, spent about $105,000 on CDs of Beethoven and had them distributed to ncw parents in the state.

Some of the musical myths are examined below.

Myth #1: Classical music makes babies smarter

No scientific experimentation has been able to substantiate the Mozart effect on children. In fact, after some years of replicated study, the Mozart effect was debunked, although studies are still ongoing. There is no good evidence that listening to Mozart or any song or sound does anything for intelligence or cognitive skills in areas that are not musical. Classical music certainly does not hurt an infant's development. If it calms the parent down, it should certainly calm the baby down as well. A research carried out by Rauscher and his colleagues in 1993 revealed that classical music had a calming effect on the participants.

Myth #2: Baby videos and visuals improve brain development

Your baby is smart and will begin to watch television at an average age of 5 months. You must have heard marketers promoting certain CDs to help develop your baby's brain, but research studies have shown contrasting results. You should know that before the age of two, watching TV can actually be detrimental to your baby's language development. Children who spent more than two hours watching television learned fewer words than those with less screen time.

It is far better for your kid to learn words from you and other adults in his/her environment than from the TV. Also, talking to kids is very good, especially when you express excitement when your child tries to vocalize the word(s) back to you.

You may want to ask why videos are not good even though kids love them. The reason is that babies have very sharp sensitivity to flashing colors. Once their attention is caught, they may cry if you try to take them away from the screen. Also, research shows that exposure of kids to violent movies or programs before the age of three will likely make your child develop ADHD. You should be cautious with this.

Myth #3: Listening to music will improve your child's intelligence quotient

There may be benefits of music for a child's brain power, but improving their intelligence quotient is not one. The fact is that musical training for your child from 4 or 5 can enhance the way they process sounds in a busy environment like a playground. The improved brain functioning may help to enhance memory and attention span, allowing your kid to focus and concentrate while in class. If your child is enrolled in music training, research also shows a benefit in improving communication skills as well.

So on your kid's academics, yes! Music may have a good and strong impact, but not on the IQ.

Myth #4: Music may not be good for my child to be successful

The truth is, even though music may not be able to boost your child's IQ, it will aid her in having greater success in life. As said by James Hudziak, a professor at the University of Vermont, training on an instrument can develop cortical organizational skill, emotional regulation, anxiety management.

It is no doubt that some kids have the innate ability to be good at some certain sports. But learning an instrument takes time, resilience and dedication. Even if he has natural musical talent, instruments are not learned in just a few attempts. Commitment to the endeavor will help him learn perseverance and how to push through for success as he goes through adolescence and adulthood.

A DIET FOR A MOTHER AND A BABY: MYTHS AND FACTS

Being a new parent is fantastic and as a new parent what you eat and what your baby eats is often a topic of discussion. As a breastfeeding mother, you are likely to have heard some opinions about what you should or should not eat. You will probably agree that from the time your baby bump started showing, you have been receiving endless advice on nutrition for both you and your baby. And since you delivered, you will have no doubt gotten even more. The truth is that findings have confirmed that allergies are the only exception to what you can eat as a nursing mother. Here are some of the myths you should be aware of concerning diet for you and your lovely baby!

Myth #1: Your baby has food allergies because you are allergic

This is false because, in reality, your trigger food may not cause a reaction in your baby. In fact, certain allergies run in families but this does not infer that because you are allergic to a food, then your baby will also be allergic to it.

Speak to your pediatrician if you notice that your child has food allergies so that you can get professional help.

Myth #2: Only a balanced diet should be eaten during breastfeeding months

A balanced diet is generally low in dietary fiber and contains every class of food in the right proportion. As said earlier, certain allergies may run in your family and in the family of your baby's father of which you may not be aware. Eating foods like that shellfish can upset your baby's stomach if he is born with an allergy to it.

Myth #3: Hyperactivity is caused by sugar in the mother's food

You may have heard this frequently, but it is not so. The question you should ask yourself is "Does the sugar I take move directly into my breast milk?" The fact is every sugar you consume gets converted even if your baby is suckling directly as you are eating. This misconception came from the research carried out by Benjamin Feingold who published that food that contains salicylates can cause hyperactivity. Research has since debunked this. In 2011, the study carried out by Yujeong and Hyeja showed that there is no correlation between the total volume of sugar intake and hyperactivity.

Myth #4: A mother should feed her baby every two hours

This myth is entirely disturbing and may traumatize you if you try it for a week. You will become tired and will not want to get pregnant again after one child. Your body system will deteriorate quickly due to the stress and lack of sleep. Do not heed to this myth. Many mothers fall for this subjective idea and feed their babies every two hours throughout the night. Though the idea stems from the view that the baby is not eating enough, you should not bother yourself.

Come to think of it, you will definitely be inconveniencing yourself and your baby doing this. One of the ways to know if your kid is not eating enough is to observe his stools each day. A good indicator is 6 wet diapers and 2 to 3 stools passed each day from age one downward.

Myth #5: Formulas are similar to breast milk

Many parents become carried away by this myth. One key thing you should understand is that your breast milk contains living cells, enzymes, and antibodies (also called hormones) and is in no way similar to formulas. Formulas are only manufactured to look like breast milk but they do not contain any living cells. Another fact is that your breast milk changes to suit perfectly your baby's changing needs but the formula is also the same. This does not mean that your child will not grow if you have no choice but to bottle-feed your child due to uncontrollable circumstances.

Myth #6: A breastfeeding mother should stop in case of a breast infection or blocked duck.

Factually, many infections are passed to a baby even before the mother is aware of them. Apart from the fact that the baby's protection depends on the breast milk from the mother, she will develop the mother's immunity for fighting the infection as well. Now, concerning a blocked duct, as a nursing mother, your duct may be blocked if you supplement your baby's food with formula. Due to the supplementation of formula or solid foods, your breasts start to have a buildup due to less frequent freeding.

The best and most natural way to unblock your duct is to breastfeed your baby as many times as possible. But once infection occurs due to your failure to breastfeed your baby as necessary, you will need antibiotics and physician consultation. But the most important part of preventing infections is to give your lovely baby as much breast milk as required. Your baby's diet is very important for healthy living. Maintain good nutrition and get your baby good nutrition, as this is the only way to have a healthy baby with a good immune and hormone system.

Part Three

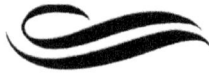

THE MAIN STAGES OF A CHILD'S DEVELOPMENT, PECULIAR BEHAVIORAL PATTERNS, AND ISSUES

Watching a child grow is indeed a beautiful thing. Only a few things delight a parent more than watching their children blossom like a tender flower into a great tree. Growth is gradual and has different phases. Each of these phases has peculiar behavioral patterns as well as its own peculiar issues. It is important that you are conversant with each of these stages and their peculiarities especially as a parent so that you can help your child grow into the kind of man or woman you will be proud of. The main stages of a child's development and the peculiar behavioral pattern and like issues that accompany each stage are all discussed in this part. These developmental and behavioral patterns as well as the issues that are peculiar to children of each age are not mere conjectures based on popular opinion; they are based on the research carried out by Louise Bates Ames, Elizabeth Crary, and other trusted sources on children. You can be sure that the information you are about to get is top quality and from credible sources.

BABY BY 1 MONTH

When you realize your baby is already a month old, it is so exciting! There are some specific development and behavioral patterns that are associated with this milestone as well as some peculiar issues.

Developments and Behavioral patterns

Below are some of the behavioral patterns to expect when your child is a month old:

Personality begins to emerge

All your baby will do in the first few weeks is sleep, eat, cry, and defecate but things begin to change gradually when the child is a month old. You will notice that your child will start cooing and this first sign that your baby is developing is often heartwarming.

Taller and bigger

The growth of your baby will also be reflected in the height and weight of the baby when the child is a month old. According to the World Health Organization (WHO), the average weight of a child at one month old 9.9 pounds. Just like adults, some babies weigh less or more. Don't be scared if your baby does not match this weight. However, if you feel that your baby is either overweight or underweight, you can always book an appointment with your pediatrician.

Growth spurt

This growth spurt does not occur when the child is exactly one month old but around six weeks. You will notice that your child will become more demanding, desiring to be fed more frequently than before. Get set for this growth spurt mentally so that you will be a happy parent of a happy child.

Better use of the five senses

Another behavioral pattern you will notice when your child is a month older is that you will observe (if you are a good observer) that your child will start having better use of the five senses. The eyes may still wander, which will make it difficult for you to determine how far your child can see. However, the child will be able to focus more on one or two objects by this age. Your child will also grow more responsive to sounds because the fluids that prevent the child from hearing well initially will have started clearing off. The child's sense of smell, as well as sensitivity to touch, will also become sharper.

Smiles

It is possible that your child will start smiling before a month but it is more likely that it will be about then. That first glow of the cheek always delights parents. If the child has been smiling before one month old, the child will start smiling more frequently when he or she is one month old. Those bright faces are moments worth living for. No amount of money can buy the happiness a happy child gives a parent.

Issues

Just as there are behavioral patterns that are often exclusive to a one-month-old baby, there are also issues that are often common at that age. These issues include:

Slow feeding

Don't be too surprised to find out that your one-month-old baby feeds slowly or has a problem with sucking. However, it is not normal and you need to talk to your health provider as fast as possible to resolve the issue before it gets out of hand.

Inability to blink when exposed to bright light

It is also a potential red flag when you notice that your one-month-old child does not blink when a bright light is flashed at him or her. It is an indicator of a sight defect, especially when you notice that it occurs consistently. Of course, see you pediatrician as soon as possible to discuss this issue in case your child has it.

Inability to respond to loud sound

If your child is also not responding to loud noises, you need to talk to your pediatrician immediately.

Inability to focus on objects

It is not like you should expect your child to focus well on objects when the child is still a month old. However, it is not a good sign when your child does not focus on any object or even follow objects with his or her eyes when the object is taken away.

Trembling jaws

When your one-month-old baby cries, it is not abnormal that the jaw trembles. However, it is not a good sign when your child's jaw trembles when the child is not crying or pumped up.

BABY BY 2 MONTHS

When your child becomes two months old, there are more activities she can participate in and you will be forgiven for wondering what has happened to that baby that slept for the most of the day. The common developmental and behavioral pattern, as well as issues associated with this milestone, are discussed below:

Developments and Behavioral patterns
Cry, cry, cry

Your child will sleep less when he or she is two months old. This will let you have more time to stimulate the baby for play and this is really nice. However, this increase in activity comes with a price: frequent crying. During this age, your baby will sleep around 15 hours daily, with nighttime accounting for about 8 hours out of that. Two-month-old babies often cry a lot. It is almost as though they have decided to sleep less so that they can cry more. They will only cry less during the evening. If you are not a patient parent, you might feel frustrated during this period. Love your baby and put up with his crying all the same. If in any case, you feel that the frequency and intensity of your baby's cry are unacceptable, you can ask your pediatrician for help.

More weight and height

It is also normal that your child will increase in weight and height when she is two months old. The average weight for two-month-old babies for boys and girls is 12.3 and 11.3 respectively. The average height for boys and girls is 23 inches and 22.5 inches respectively. These averages are based on the specification of the World Health Organization (WHO). As stated earlier, babies vary in height and weight; hence, don't worry unnecessarily if your baby does not meet these averages. There are various factors that determine the height and weight of babies. Always talk to your pediatrician when you need any clarification.

The five senses

The development of your child at two months old is quite obvious. You will notice that she will be able to not just focus on more objects but also able to follow objects with her eyes even when the object is moved a full 180 degrees! Your child will also be able to observe more colors rather than just black and white. You can take advantage of this to show the child more colorful patterns to help the child further develop his or her vision.

You will also be able to have a better conversation with your child at this stage because the child will be able to listen more actively. The child will not only listen but also respond by cooing. You can also find the child moving his or her arms and legs to respond to the things you are saying to him or her during this milestone. You will also find your child responding more to touches and display a sign of enjoying your touch and warmth at this stage.

Stronger baby

Your baby will be stronger at this stage and ready for more play. He will be able to lift his or her shoulders during tummy time at this stage of his or her life. The child will also be able to lift up his head while sitting. The muscles of the neck are stronger now and this offers the child the opportunity to turn his neck to an extent.

Coordinated movement

The movement of your two-month-old child will also be more coordinated and less jerky at this milestone. This is because the child will have better control of her muscles at this stage. Don't be surprised if the child begins trying out new positions that she has never tried before at this stage. The awareness of the baby is better and she will play better at this phase. You can even find the child trying to make herself happy by sucking her thumb when the child is two months old.

Commons issues associated with two-month-old babies

Below are common issues that are common to babies who are two months old:

Teething: Most babies do not begin teething at two months old but you cannot rule out the possibility. In case you notice that your baby is crying often, drooling and unable to sleep well, it might be a result of teething. Don't hesitate to talk to your pediatrician so that your child can receive adequate help as soon as possible.

Coughing: Another common issue associated with two months old is coughing. One of the most common reasons for coughing for babies of this age is cold. Treat your child on time when you notice this.

Diarrhea: If you realize that the poop of your two-month-old baby is more watery than usual, it is most likely a sign of diarrhea. You need to arrange for the treatment of the child as soon as possible. Call your pediatrician for help.

Constipation: How you will be able to know that your baby is constipated is when you notice that the poop of your baby is more like hard balls with a corresponding hard belly.

Oversleeping: Another health concern for two-month-old babies is when they sleep for most of the day. This may not necessarily indicate a problem but it can mean that something is not right. If you notice that your baby sleeps for more than 16 hours a day consistently, it might be a sign of sickness. Speak to your pediatrician about the concern as fast as possible.

Staying awake more than usual: In the same way that it is not good for your child to be passive for a prolonged period of time, it is not also good if your child is awake for a large part of the day. Call the attention of your pediatrician if you are not sure your child is healthy.

BABY BY 3 MONTHS

Most parents perceive the third month as an enchanted month because the baby still sleeps for a considerable period of the day, especially at night, and still depends on you for mobility. This lack of independence in terms of mobility makes the child incapable of giving you much stress. With little mischief to make, your little cutie is a delight at this age. Things to look out for, in terms of development, behavioral pattern, and issues that are particular to this milestone are discussed below:

Development and behavioral pattern peculiar to three-month-old babies

Laugh out loud

Before your child is three months old, he or she will smile predominantly but the story changes when the child is three months old. You will find your baby being able to laugh out loud when he or she is tickled or finds a gesture to be funny.

Higher anticipation

Your baby will also have better response and anticipation in this milestone. You will find him or her lifting up his or her hand in response to your gesture to carry him or her. The child will also be able to roll over and will respond to sounds faster than you have observed before.

Sign of coordinated speech

The moment most parents wait for is when their baby starts stringing together some vowels compared to the mere cooing sounds that the child makes before he is three months old. Get set to be blown away in this enchanted month as your baby begins to show signs of being able to speak coherently. Don't expect too much. Your child will be a better speaker in the next few months.

Toy freak

Your baby will be able to play with sensory toys at this stage. Toys that are designed to play music when the child moves them are often favorites. You will observe that your child will find happiness squeaking and rattling such toys because he or she has gotten accustomed to the nice sound the toy makes.

Weight and height

I am sure you expect your baby to grow taller and bigger at this age. The average weight for boys is 14.1 pounds while that of girls is 12.9. The average length is also different for both boy and girls. It is 24.2 inches for boys while girls are 23.5 inches. Your baby might be a little taller or shorter than this average or even weigh more or less than this average but as long as your baby is growing healthily, there is no cause for alarm.

Expect a growth spurt in this milestone which will make your baby more hungry than usual. This growth spurt is short-lived; so give your child everything he or she demands from you, be it be food or more attention during this period. Always talk to your pediatrician if you feel your child is not growing as much as it should be for a three-month-old.

No more clenched fists

At three months old, your child will open and close his hands more. The days of a consistent clenched fist is over! The baby will also be able to use his arms to support himself as he raises his head during tummy time. It is better to let the baby play on the floor during this age because there is the tendency of the baby to swing at things.

Sleep

The sleep pattern of a three-month-old is similar to a two-month-old's. They sleep for about 15 hours daily, mostly at night. Avoid getting the child tired because you will be surprised to find that a tired baby does not sleep readily. It is advised that you keep the room dark and cool to stimulate your baby to sleep. Some babies will still not sleep even after this but most babies will sleep when the conditions are right.

Common issues associated with three-month-old babies

Common issues commonly found among babies in this milestone include:

Poor response to loud sound

Your baby has a relatively good grasp of the five senses when he or she is three months old. So it is an anomaly when you observe that your baby is not responding when loud sounds are blared at him or her. It is also not normal that you speak to your child and the child does not respond to the sound of your voice at this age. Your pediatrician should know about that.

The child doesn't pay attention to new faces

You also need to talk to your pediatrician when you realize that your child cannot distinguish between your face and that of strangers or members of your family the baby has never seen before.

Your child doesn't push down with her feet when you hold her upright or place her on a flat surface

This is often common among three-month-old babies and it should bother you when you have a baby that is passive in this regard.

Consistently not following objects with the eyes

It is also not normal if your child is not following objects with his eyes. The use of the senses expected at this milestone makes it something you need to be concerned about when you notice that the eyes of your baby stay glued to a particular spot when objects are being moved to and fro right in front of him.

Refusal to smile

Of course, your baby will not smile every time. However, it is also not good if your child repeatedly does not smile when funny gestures are made toward her. Smiling is a common theme when your child is three months old. It may be a sign of being sick and you need to see your pediatrician to allay any fear as soon as possible.

The incapacity to hold or grasp objects

Your three-month-old baby is expected to be able to hold objects and play with them. It is not normal for your child to have difficulty holding or grabbing objects. Contact your pediatrician immediately so that any sickness can be diagnosed and treated as soon as possible.

Not moving objects or hands toward the mouth

Parents are often advised to be sure that their child doesn't put things that can be harmful to their health in their mouth. However, it is not normal if your child does not make attempts to move his hand or objects toward his mouth. Talk to your pediatrician as soon as possible.

Baby's eyes still seem closed most of the time

You should not observe that your three-month-old has her eyes closed for most of the day. As said earlier, your child should have relatively good use of her eyes by this point. Therefore, talk to your pediatrician if you notice your child often keeps her eyes closed.

Your child doesn't babble

The happy sound of a babbling child brings delight to the heart of the parents. Not babbling can be a sign of a speech inhibition.

BABY BY 5 MONTHS

Wow! It's five months already. There are lots of beautiful moments when your precious princess or little Prince Charming is five months old. Guess what? Expect to hear a "Dada" or "Mama" in this enchanting milestone. You will feel like some kind of super coach and parenting begins to really feel like an amazing journey! Let me take you through the developmental and behavioral as well as particular issues that come with your baby turning five months.

The developmental and behavioral pattern associated with five-month-old babies
Height and weight

Your baby is growing bigger and taller at five months old and the days of holding a tiny cutie are gone. Your baby on average will weigh 16.6 pounds if he is a boy but you can expect an average weight of 15.2 pounds for a girl. You can be sure that your baby has no growth deficiency when he gains at least a pound per month. Any irregular or stagnant growth should be reported to your pediatrician as fast as you can.

Use of the five senses

The use of the five senses of a five-month-old child is way better than when the child was younger. Your baby will be able to distinguish between different colors better than she used to do before getting to this milestone. Normally before now, the child will only be able to distinguish bold or bright colors but the story becomes different when the child turns five months. You can also expect a better response to sound at this stage of your baby's life. She will turn to you faster and listen to you with rapt attention. Isn't that amazing?

Speech

Your baby's speech will become better at this stage too. You will observe him repeating the sounds you make. He can even repeat them continuously. Those moments are often delightful, especially the first time.

Use of the hands

Your baby will have a better grip and will be seen bringing both hands together to amuse herself. You will find her reaching out for objects with both hands and grasping them with the full use of all the fingers.

A better understanding of existence

You five-month-old will learn that objects that are not in his or her vicinity can still exist. Get set to see your baby keep objects and show them again while playing.

Roll over time

Expect your child to start rolling over when he reaches this age. It is also not out of place to see your child sway from one side to the other. Some babies begin to roll over at four months. If your child is not rolling over by five months, you don't need to be panicky. However, if you notice that there are no changes to that when the child is six months, you need to let your pediatrician be aware of the situation.

Crawling

It is true that most babies don't start crawling until they are six months and some will not even start until they are ten months. So, don't get worked up about it if you observe that your five-month-old baby is not yet crawling. However, don't be surprised if you notice that your baby begins to crawl when he or she reaches this milestone. It reflects that your baby has a determined personality. That should definitely make you glad!

Solid food

Most babies are able to take solid food when they are five months old. Ensure you discuss with your pediatrician before you make the decision to start your baby on solid food. If your pediatrician approves this, ensure you don't rush the process. Introduce it to the child slowly and notice his or her response.

Less sleep

Sleep regression is common at this stage. Your baby's brain is more active now and she will not sleep as deeply as she used to. Don't be too perturbed, because this will not last more than six weeks. You can always speak to your pediatrician if you feel your child has an irregular sleep schedule.

Common issues associated with five-month-old babies

The common issues you may have to deal with when your child is five months old are:

- ❖ Teething
- ❖ Irregular pooping
- ❖ Constipation
- ❖ Diarrhea
- ❖ Cough
- ❖ Vomiting
- ❖ Fever
- ❖ Stuffy nose

Once you notice that your baby is battling any of these issues, don't try to do something you aren't sure will work. Your baby should be far too precious to you for risky and careless experiments. Your pediatrician has been trained to help you handle such issues. You will be making a smart choice by speaking to him or her to get professional services.

BABY BY 6 MONTHS

Your baby is half a year old! It is so incredible to realize that your baby is just six months away from being a year old! She will begin to show an amazing repertoire of skills when she reaches this milestone. Expect your child to cry when someone else picks her up at this stage. Below are the peculiar developmental, behavioral, and specific problems that you might encounter as your child reaches this age.

Developmental and behavioral patterns

Height and weight

I am sure you are curious to find out how your six-month-old baby will weigh and how tall he will be. On average, your six-month-old will weigh 16.1 pounds as a girl and 17.5 pounds as a boy. For height, expect your boy to be 26.6 inches and your girl to be 25.9 inches on the average. Remember that all babies are not the same. Watch for a steady growth rate rather than hitting an average. If you are not confident about the growth rate of your baby, speak to your pediatrician for an expert view.

Growth spurt

Your six-month-old can become crankier than usual and the reason for this could easily be a growth spurt. The good news is that this will only last for a few days and normalcy will be restored again.

The five senses

The taste bud of your six-month-old is now developed such that the baby can distinguish between different tastes. Don't be surprised if she has a favorite food at this stage. Your baby will also have good control of the use of her eyes. She will be able to look at you as you move across the room with ease. Your child will not only look at objects but will be able to examine them closely. Don't be too surprised to see her pay closer attention to her toys when she reaches this milestone. She may carry out this examination with her mouth and that is why you need to ensure that you don't allow your six-month-old to play with objects that may harm her when she puts them into her mouth.

Your child will also be able to respond faster to sounds around him. A fascinating part of the use of the five senses for your six-month-old baby is that he will begin to be able to notice that the voices of people are not the same. Your voice will sound more distinct to him when he reaches this milestone. You will notice your child touching objects to examine the differences in their texture. This experiment with textures may be carried out also with his body parts.

Speech

Your six-month-old will also speak better. He will be able to say a few consonants and you can expect a lot of bababababababa or dadadadadada as the child gets to this milestone. The way your baby laughs and giggles will also change when the child is six months old. The laugh will be louder and the giggles will be more pronounced. If you are a good comedian, you have a ready-made audience in your baby at this stage.

Rollover

Your baby will have been rolling over before she reaches this milestone. The major difference here is that she will be able to roll in both directions now. Get set to be amused as your baby rolls front to back and back to front.

Stronger arm

Your baby will be able to hold small objects and even pull them to himself when he is six months old. He will be able to sit up but you might need to help in some ways. Don't be surprised to also see your child moving objects from one hand to the other.

Solid food

Most six-month-olds are ready for solid food. However, it is always safer to talk to your pediatrician about this before you decide to start feeding solid food to your baby. Once your pediatrician approves your plan, you can start feeding your baby with solid food but you should observe the way she reacts as you do the feeding. Do it slowly till your baby shows that she is at home with the food.

Common issues

Teething

Teething is a major concern for parents of six-month-old babies. The symptoms of teething are more frequent crying or swollen gums. Teething will also make the child drool and be unable to sleep with ease. If you also notice that your baby will not accept a bottle, it can be a symptom of teething. Your pediatrician is your best option once you notice these symptoms.

Other issues that are common to six-month-old babies include:

- ❖ Irregular pooping
- ❖ Constipation

- ❖ Diarrhea
- ❖ Cough
- ❖ Fever

Your pediatrician should know in case you notice that your six-month-old bay is having to deal with any of these issues.

BABY BY 8 MONTHS

Your eight-month-old baby will have an incredible awareness of himself as well as an impressive awareness of his environment. A distinctive feature of this milestone is that your baby does not want to separate from you at any time. He may cry and have separation anxiety whenever you are not around. This should not bother you because it actually shows that there is a good bond between the two of you. In the event that you have to leave your child with caregivers, the separation anxiety will not be a serious issue because the caregivers will be able to stop your baby from crying shortly after you are gone. The distinguishing developmental and behavioral patterns are rolled out here. There are also issues that pertain to this milestone and they are also discussed below.

Developmental and behavioral patterns

Weight and height

The World Health Organization posits that on average, your eight-month-old girl should weigh 17.5 pounds and a boy 19.0 pounds. The average height for boys is 27.8 inches while the average height for girls is 27.1 inches. Never forget that your focus should not be on the average but the fact that your child has a steady growth rate. Any suspicion of growth deficiency should be reported to your pediatrician.

Use of the five senses

Expect a better use of the five senses from your eight-month-old baby. Your baby will not only be able to see close things better but will be able to identify objects across the room. This improved sight will make your child go for objects and grab them to play with them. Eight-month-old babies often find textures fascinating and this is reflected in how they love to touch tags and handles to feel the differences in their textures.

Sitting

Your eight-month-old baby will be able to sit by himself but watch out because she might still need your assistance once in a while. This assistance is pertinent because she will want to lean over to pick up toys and will need your help to avoid tumbling over and getting hurt.

Variety of movements

When your baby reaches this milestone, he will have a number of movements up his sleeves. You will find him crouching, rolling, and twisting. It is also not out of place to find your baby rocking while kneeling. All of these movements are foundations upon which the moment you have been waiting for will be built—acrawling!

Preparation for crawling

Some babies start crawling when they are eight months old, but this is more of an exception rather than the rule. What happens most of the time when your child is eight months old is to prepare him or herself for crawling. You will find your baby scooting or rolling around in order to move to his or her destination. It is not an anomaly if your baby does not crawl at all because some babies start walking without crawling.

Feeding

Unless otherwise stated by your pediatrician, your eight-month-old baby will be able to eat solid food comfortably, but that does not stop you from still feeding the child with formula as well as breastfeeding. In fact, the major source of nutrition for eight-month-olds remains fluids. You can train your child with a sippy cup at this age. Introduce it to her more like a toy to play with initially. Babies like to put objects to their mouth, so you may not even need to bring the sippy cup to her mouth before she does that by herself. This training is important because it will help your child start drinking from a cup easier and faster.

Sleep pattern

At eight months, your child is growing and this growth will lead to less sleep. Your baby will no longer sleep up to 15 hours. When he reaches this milestone, he will not sleep more than 10 or 12 hours a day in the worst-case scenario. Typically, your baby will need two naps as well as three and a half hours of sleep in the daytime. Don't be surprised to find that your baby wakes up in the night more than you are accustomed to when he is eight months old. You can find him trying to pull himself up.

You need to be prepared for this as a working mom because your baby is most likely going to wake up to spend more time with you in the night to make up for the lost time in the afternoon when you left her with caregivers. Be patient and learn more skills that can put a baby to sleep to avoid being stressed out. Sleep training is not as easy as it sounds but if you are able to successfully sleep-train your child, it will be beneficial to both of you. This is because, whenever you baby wakes up in the night, she will not need your help to go back to sleep. The resultant effect of that is more sleep for both of you.

Common issues

The particular health concerns that are often associated with being eight months old are:

- ❖ Constipation
- ❖ Diarrhea
- ❖ Vomiting
- ❖ Fever

There is only one solution you should think about when you notice any of these issues and it is to speak to your pediatrician. Don't give your child any medication without the guidance of your pediatrician because it can be very risky for the health of your baby.

BABY BY 10 MONTHS

Oh my God! It is ten months already! You will find yourself exclaiming this because you will remember vividly how you went through the labor and the early days of your baby and it all felt like yesterday. Your baby will soon become a toddler and will be more demanding, but it is all worth it because you have someone you can show genuine affection and who will be able to replicate. Your baby will be quite independent at this age and will need you to pay more attention to him to avoid a situation where the child hurts himself. I know you are looking forward to the development, behavior, and problems that children who are ten months old exhibit. Here you are!

Developmental and behavioral patterns
Height and weight

Wondering how tall your ten-month-old baby will be? The gender of your baby determines this. On the average, your baby girl will be 28.1 inches tall while your baby boy will be 28.9 inches tall. The weight of your child will also vary based on the gender. Your baby boy on the average will weigh 20.2 pounds while your baby girl will weigh 18.7 pounds. Just like I have always told you about the height and weight of babies, don't get carried away by averages.

It should be more important to you that your child is growing steadily. Never forget also that you need to report any case of stunted growth to your pediatrician. You will be able to either get an assurance that there is no cause for alarm or know what needs to be done to help your child grow. Mind you, it is not only cases of stunted growth that should be reported to your doctor. You should also let your pediatrician be aware of excessive weight. Babies with excessive weight are likely going to be obese by age three. Don't throw caution to the wind.

It is also important to know that growth is not automatic. You have an important role to play in ensuring that your baby grows as expected of a ten-month-old. A huge part of this is to feed your baby well. Your ten-month-old will be able to eat solid food but you should never forget that the child needs milk daily. You should still maintain the habit of giving your baby formula and breastfeeding. You have a responsibility to watch over your child, especially in the early years before she is able to look after herself. You need to be dutiful in your approach to parenting.

The five senses

Your ten-month-old will be able to respond to sounds admirably but that is not all. He will be able to differentiate between sounds. He will be able to tell when you are speaking or if it's someone else. He will also be able to tell when the doorbell is ringing or if music is playing. Sounds will no longer startle the child because he will be able to tell the difference between important sounds and ones that should be ignored. That is impressive, isn't it?

Your baby will also be able to tell that her toys that produce sounds don't have the same sound. For example, if your baby has a rattle, she will know that she needs to shake it to get the distinctive sound. She will be know if she needs to push the buttons on a toy to make it produce the desired sound. Your child will start displaying a good level of intelligence, which makes her ready to learn basic things in this milestone.

Independent sitting

Unlike the milestones before now, your baby will be able to sit without any support when he is ten months old. This independent sitting gives you peace of mind because you can be sure that he will not stumble or fall without your attention. This means you can have your baby sit down while you go about your activities. Of course, this does not mean that you should not observe the baby periodically just because he or she is sitting down because of the next behavioral and developmental pattern to be discussed: crawling.

Crawling

Most babies crawl before they are ten months old but it is not a problem if your baby just begins to crawl now. Never forget that your baby does not have to crawl. She can start standing and walking without crawling, so there is no cause for alarm. However, if it is important to you that your baby crawls, you can put her favorite toy out of her reach and encourage her to get it.

Standing

Most ten-month-old babies are able to stand, though they might need to hold on to something to keep from falling. You can expect your baby to do the same when he reaches this milestone.

Excellent use of the hands

Your ten-month-old baby will be able to make good use of his or her hands to do some impressive things. You will find her being able to point to things she finds fascinating. All the fingers are no longer treated as the same. Isn't this exciting?

Speech

Your baby will no longer blab and will be able to call you Mama or Dada at this age. It is always satisfying to hear this, especially the first time. It makes you feel every sacrifice has been worth it. It is almost as though your child is saying, "Thank you for being there for me all this while." Your child will not only say dada and mama all day long;

he will be able to say a few other words as well when he gets to this milestone.

Independent feeding

Your ten-month-old baby will be able to feed himself at this age. So it should not be strange to you that your baby is able to use the bottle to feed himself or help himself to some little chops. Your baby might begin to crave new food ideas at this stage. Mind you, this newfound independence does not in any way exempt you from watching over him, as he might not be able to handle the feeding well, which may lead to choking. I am sure you don't want that, so don't be so excited by your baby beginning to act like a little adult that you leave him alone without keeping an eye on him. As earlier stated, your child also needs milk. The fact that your child is able to feed himself with little support from you does not take the place of breastfeeding the child at this stage of his life.

Sleep pattern

The pattern of sleep common to ten-month-old babies is a big relief for the parents. This is because ten-month-olds often have two naps during the day and can sleep as much as eleven to twelve hours at night without waking up. Therefore, you can sleep more at night now than when your baby was eight months when she would wake up in the night and demand that you lure her back to sleep before got yours.

Common issues

The following issues are peculiar to babies who are ten months old:

- ❖ Diarrhea
- ❖ Constipation
- ❖ Coughing
- ❖ Vomiting
- ❖ Fever
- ❖ Teething pain

Just like every other milestone, your ten-month-old baby should be taken to your pediatrician for quick attention when you notice that he or she is suffering from any of the above issues. Teething pain in particular will make you child reject the bottle and not feed well. You need to take action as soon as possible. Never assume that any of these issues is minimal or something you can just gloss over. These issues can be a symptom of a more harmful disease. Your pediatrician is always your safest bet.

BABY BY 12 MONTHS

Your little baby is a year old! How satisfying and interesting this feeling is for parents. You probably want to throw a birthday party to mark this milestone. Don't hold back; your baby deserves it. Of course, the birthday party should not cut too deep into your budget because you still have a lot of expenses to incur as your child grows older. That aside, it is a milestone worth celebrating. Your baby has not been walking before now or has been walking with support? That is about to change! Are you set? Let's get down to the developmental and behavioral patterns as well as issues that are common to babies when they reach this milestone.

Developmental and behavioral patterns
Weight and height

A healthy child should be growing at a steady rate now, adding about half an inch each month to his height and three or more ounces to his weight per week. One-year-olds will weigh 21.3 pound for boys and 21.9 pounds for girls on average. Regarding height, on average, your baby boy should be 29.8 inches and your baby girl should be 29.1 inches. In general, your baby is likely to be ten inches taller than he was when you first gave birth to him.

The five senses

People need to be careful concerning gossiping about you around your child now because she can pick up sounds more accurately than before. Her hearing is quite good now and she can pay rapt attention when you speak and the quick rate of response will convince you of how well your child can now hear you. Get set to do a lot more reading to your child now because she will be able to look and listen at the same time now. Your one-year-old will also be able to react to sensations faster now. She will feel like touching more objects as she clocks one year just for the sake of noting the differences in the texture of various objects.

Distinguishing of familiar and strange faces

Your baby will also be affectionate toward you and his caregivers but will be anxious to see strange faces but will not want to be carried by them.

Motor skills

Your one-year-old baby will have a better mastery of motor skills. You will find your baby holding out his hand when you are trying to dress him. It is also not out of place to find your baby walking upstairs at this stage of development. Pincer grasp, which involves using the thumb and one finger to pick up an object like raisins, will also be displayed by your baby at this stage of development. Poking, pointing, and pinching are also common for babies of this age. Your baby will be able to put objects into a bucket and remove them again while playing. Scribbling with a marker or crayon is also not impossible for your baby when he is a year old. You can also find your child pointing to his own nose, ears, eyes, or head.

Sitting

Your baby would have mastered the art of sitting by this age. She will be able to sit for a long period of time without your assistance. That should be good news to you because your baby is pretty able to look after herself now and that will make you able to concentrate on other things without being too worried about her. He or she will be able to reach out, twisting and turning with ease.

Standing

Most babies are able to stand without support when they reach this milestone for a while before they sit back again. Expect this development for your baby as well.

Walking

A number of toddlers start walking when they are a year old and it is not unusual to see your child begin to take his or her first steps at this age. However, if your child is not walking by the time he reaches this milestone, don't be bothered unless you suspect that his growth is stunted. Your suspicion should be reported to your pediatrician and not acted upon out of curiosity or fear. Some babies will not walk until they are close to one and a half years old. There is no cause for alarm.

Talking

Expect more dada and mama at this stage of your child's development. More combination of syllables will also be seen as the child begins to gradually acquire a better grip of language.

Comprehension

Your one-year-old baby will display better comprehension of your instructions at this age and this will be confirmed by the way he or she responds to your commands. Simple instructions that involve just one step like picking up a toy or looking at a book will be obeyed by your child at this stage of her development. Her cognitive skills will be a little advanced and that will make her capable of realizing the use of objects commonly found in your home like a spoon, phone, or toothbrush. She will also be able to recognize the correlation between words uttered by you and the images you show her in a book. Familiar songs or stories will also catch the attention of your growing child and she will react to them.

Emotions

Your baby will also be fond of expressing his or her emotions in peculiar ways when he reaches this milestone. He will express happiness, frustration, and sadness with various sounds or cries that will pass across his message to you. Frustration can make your one-year-old react with tantrums in protestation of not being treated in the way he desires. He will also be able to shake his head to say no. You will find your child smiling or laughing when playing or when he finds something that amuses him.

Curiosity

Don't be surprised when you notice that your child is quite experimental at this stage of her life. She can throw her cup to the ground just to find out what happens.

Feeding

There will be a shift in the feeding pattern of your baby as he clocks one year. He will eat more now, taking three meals daily and two or three snacks in addition to the breast milk or formula you give him daily. His appetite will increase considerably but you don't have to worry too much about this because it will drop in the next few months. He will know to stop when he is full, so don't bother yourself about that. Your child will also be able to eat with a spoon at this stage but he might still be quite clumsy. You can always report any case of abnormal eating to your pediatrician.

Sleep pattern

Your child will sleep an average of 13 to 14 hours when she gets to this milestone. Of those, 10 to 11 will be at night. Expect the child to take two to three naps equivalent to two to three hours during the afternoon. You can be confident of having your night's rest without disturbances and interruptions when your child is a year old. Any irregular sleeping pattern should be reported to your pediatrician as soon as possible.

Issues

Common health concerns peculiar to one-year-olds are:

Colds

One-year-old children often contract colds at least once in a month. Fluids and rest are recommended for such situations but if you notice that he situation is getting out of hand, speak to your pediatrician as soon as possible.

Conjunctivitis

This is an infection that affects the eyelids and eyeball. It might be a result of bacteria or virus. It can also be a reaction to an allergy. The eyes of the child will be sore, red, sticky, and puffy. If the conjunctivitis was caused by an allergy, it won't be contagious, but it will be if it was caused by bacteria or virus. Speak to your pediatrician right away to diagnose the type of conjunctivitis the child has and also appropriate treatment.

Asthma

Asthma is typified by a whistling wheeze when the child breathes out. It can also manifest as the child being short of breath, especially during physical activities or when resting. The child can demonstrate symptoms such as drowsiness, seizures, unresponsive breathing, and pale or blue skin. When you see these symptoms, don't hesitate, because this can affect the child more than you can imagine later on. Talk to your pediatrician immediately so that a management plan for the child can be given to you so that you can help your child cope.

Allergies

When allergens (substances in the environment) affect your child enough to cause a reaction in the child's immune system, what results is an allergy. These allergens are not substances that are harmful to every person and they include dust mites, animal furs, pollen, some foods, and insect stings. However, children with allergies react when in contact with these allergens. In case you are not sure how to handle the allergy of your child or you don't know exactly what the child is reacting to, then it is always best to speak to your doctor.

Warts

These are small growths that have the color of the flesh. They often grow on the hands of children. Warts often spread and that is why you need to ensure that your child does not pick them or chew them. Interestingly, they don't cause the child any pain but they affect the appearance of the skin. They can also appear on the face or even genitals, where they can become red and painful. See your pediatrician to handle this issue and to help your child retain her youthful and fresh skin.

BABY BY 2 YEARS

Incredible, isn't it? Your child is growing bigger and taller in what has been an amazing journey in the last two years. Both you and your child are growing and learning together.

You are getting to understand your child better and your child is getting to understand you because he can interpret what you tell him and can respond better now. Your bundle of laughter at age two has interesting developmental attributes. There are also behaviors and issues that are particular to children when they reach this milestone.

Developmental and behavioral patterns
Height and weight

Babies are not the same and they have different heights and weights even when they are the same age. The fact that your baby is bigger or taller than other children does not mean something is wrong with your child. In the same way, it is not wrong to have a child who is smaller or shorter than others. Based on the average weight of children who are two years old by the World Health Organization, your two-year-old should be 26.5 pounds as a girl and 27.5 pounds for a boy. When it comes to height, girls on average should be 33.5 inches tall and boys 34.2 inches. The most important thing is to have a child that is growing based on a healthy upward curve. However, if you are not certain that your two-year-old child is growing the way he or she ought to be, don't hesitate to call your pediatrician.

Motor skills

Your child will have a better footing as he or she walks around now. In other words, your two-year-old will be able to walk without needing support from you. Most two-year-old children can climb onto furniture by themselves and get down too without the assistance of others. Walking up the stairs will also be done with relative ease at this stage of development. Your child will not only walk, he or she may even jump with both feet at the same that. Isn't that fascinating? I am sure you can't wait to see your child performing this wonder. Two-year-olds are often fond of pulling their toys behind them while walking. It is also no secret that some are able to pull multiple toys with them.

She will be able to kick a ball when she reaches this milestone. You need to watch your two-year-old carefully because she has a tendency to run. Don't be shocked to also see your child scribble spontaneously at this age. A lot of two-year-olds also have the capacity to turn out the contents of a container. With improved motor skills, your child at this milestone can be found building a tower of four blocks and some children can even do more than that. Your child might also start having a preference when it comes to the usage of his hands at this stage. In other words, you may find him using either his left or right hand more now.

Speech

Two-year-old children are often able to use as many as fifty to a hundred words. They can even be found saying phrases of two words. However, it is important to note that not all children who are two years old display this level of proficiency of speech. Relax if you observe that your darling child is not able to speak as much as this. You can always meet with your pediatrician to discuss this if you are not certain that your child is speaking as much as he or she should be.

Teething

Though this often makes the child uncomfortable, at age two, your child's upper second molars pull through. This makes the child more effective in eating solid food.

Toilet training

A two-year-old child has the necessary awareness of herself as well as her environment to make toilet training feasible. You will be able to see that your child is ready for toilet training when you find the child letting you know she needs her diaper changed. You can also find her pulling down her pants when she needs to ease herself, showing readiness to use the potty. It is, however, important to note that you should not put undue pressure on your child at this age because some children are not able to get accustomed to using the potty until they are almost three years old.

Tantrums

This is the age when your child will be prone to tantrums. I don't mean to scare you, but you need to be ready for this. What will help you during this milestone is how well you understand your child. A proper understanding of your child will help you know what to do to stop your child when he begins to throw tantrums. For some children, all they need is something to distract them while some require shushing. Experience will teach you what works best for your child because all children are not the same. Watch your child over time and you will know what to do. Don't use the technique people around you use for their kids because it may not work for yours.

Separation anxiety

Your two-year-old will not want you out of his sight. Don't be too emotional at this stage because your child will definitely cry, but let the child understand gradually that his tears are not enough to make you change your decision. However, always assure the child about your return. It is not absurd to tell your child when you will be back exactly. Say goodbye as fast as you can and ensure you keep to your word by coming back to your sweet little one when you said you are going to return. This builds trust and a stronger bond between child and mother.

Feelings

When kids reach this milestone, they tend to be a bundle of emotions. Your greatest challenge at this stage of the life of your child is being able to stay patient and understand the emotion of the child rather than being frustrated and letting it out on your child. The truth is, it is easier said than done but once you pass this test, you will always know how to get through to your child during her difficult moments in the future. Sometimes your child is angry and is acting funny or feeling sad and could just cry and refuse to eat or play. You need to teach your child to express her emotions with words and things will be easier from that point on. Don't worry, you can handle it; you are cut out for this.

Issues

Below are some of the issues your two-year-old child might have that will require you to act quickly to avoid any developmental crisis in the future:

Does not understand the function of common tools at home like spoons, phone, fork, etc.

Has issues with imitating commons words he hears daily

- ❖ Does not have the capacity to comprehend one-word instructions
- ❖ Finds it difficult to push a wheeled toy
- ❖ Inability to walk
- ❖ Issues with speaking at least fifteen words

❖ Unable to use two-word phrases

Major health concerns include:

❖ Diarrhea

❖ Constipation

❖ Throwing up

❖ Fever

Your pediatrician should know about these issues as soon as possible to avert further problems that can complicate the health of your child.

BABY BY 3 YEARS

Happy birthday! Your child is three years old! This milestone is fascinating in the sense that your child will become more independent, which is good news for you. Your child is ready to learn because he is smarter now. He will be very curious about everything and will want you to explain everything. I need to warn you that the child will be more demanding now, but it is also fun. You survived the other milestones and this won't be different. So enjoy the ride!

Developmental and behavioral patterns
Height and weight

I am sure that you expect your three-year-old child to weigh more and have a higher height in comparison with when the child was two years old. Well, your guess is right. On the average, your three-year-old boy will weigh 31.8 pounds while your three-year-old girl will weigh 30.7 pounds. Just as I have always reminded you all through this journey, don't be concerned about meeting the average. In other words, don't stress because your child is below or above this average. As long as your child's growth is at a steady increase on a growth chart, be contented.

As regards height, on the average, your three-year-old boy will be 37.5 inches tall while your three-year-old girl will be 37.1 inches tall. I am sure you expect me to tell you that these averages are based on the recommendations of the World Health Organization, but you are wrong. These averages are based on the recommendations of the US Centers for Disease Control. Never forget that your pediatrician should be aware of any case of stunted growth, either real or perceived.

Speech

Your three-year-old will have a relatively impressive mastery of three- or four-word phrases and sentences and able to combine a variety of words to express herself. Most three-year-olds have a vocabulary of around five hundred words, among which her most frequently used words will be asking questions like why. However, if you notice that your three-year-old child is unable to speak well and stutters once in a while, it does not necessarily mean that the child has speech issues. He might simply be coming to grips with his use of language. You can always talk to your pediatrician if you are not satisfied with the progress your child is making in the way he speaks. Your fears will be allayed if they are unfounded and solutions can be offered for any speech issues if they are there.

Motor Skills

Running and walking should come to your three-year-old child with relative ease. Climbing stairs with minimal support and jumping will also be a common feature at this stage of life. Your baby has lost more baby fat at this stage and now has stronger muscles, which allows her to be ready for more physical activities. The agility of the child is better now and she can even catch a ball. Your child will get more fascinated with manipulating papers and making use of tools like crayons and finger-paint. You will also find your child being able to bend down and not fall on getting to this milestone.

Toilet training

Your child is more equipped for toilet training at this stage than when he was two. However, it is still no easy feat to be able to achieve potty-training for a three-year-old child. Your child might stay dry for most of the day but will most likely still bed-wet at night. It is normal for three-year-olds to bed-wet, so don't be overly concerned. Invest in some nighttime training pants.

Tantrums

If you think your baby had tantrums when she was two, then you will be amazed when the child is three. Most times, she will have a clear idea of what she wants to do but does not have the capacity to get it done yet. She will be frustrated by that and start crying and sometimes you are at sea about what to do. Just like when she was two years old, you need to be patient with her and try to understand her more so that you can help her. Help your child accomplish her goals such as building a giant block tower as much as you can and you will have more peace at home. I am not painting this as something simple but it is not impossible to achieve.

Separation anxiety

Your three-year-old child will want to be around you most times and will cry if you have to leave him with your relatives or drop him at school. It is normal that you will not want to see him cry, but you must not allow your emotions to make you do what you should not do. Always assure your child that you will be back in no time and keep your word. You are leaving him for a while for a noble cause and that is why you should keep the goodbye short and sweet.

Misbehavior and discipline

If you are not mentally prepared for the misbehaviors that are predominant with kids when they are three years old, you may begin to think that you have given birth to a monster. You can find your child biting someone or hitting someone at this age. Don't be too bothered; your child is simply acting three. You need to make it clear to her that such behaviors are not acceptable and you should apply punishment that is appropriate to three-year-olds when the child repeatedly misbehaves. Three-year-olds don't stop misbehaving quickly, so you need to be ready to repeatedly correct your child. However, never allow the misbehavior of your child to affect your love for her. You need to love your child unconditionally no matter what happens.

Sleep patterns

Three-year-olds often sleep between 10 to 13 hours daily. Most only have one- or two-hour naps during the afternoon, so don't be surprised if your child is so active that he will not sleep at all during the day sometimes. Three-year-old children sleep mostly at night. Putting your three-year-old to sleep is not easy, but it is achievable. Ensure you mean it when you tell your child that you will only sing one more song for him before he sleeps.

Feeding

Your three-year-old can eat virtually the same food everybody in the family eats. The major difference is that your child will eat smaller portions.

Issues

The common issues prevalent with three-year-old children include:

- ❖ Diarrhea
- ❖ Constipation
- ❖ Throwing up
- ❖ Cough
- ❖ Fever

Your pediatrician should be aware of any of this for quick treatment. Any hesitation will not help you and your child in any way.

CHILDREN UNDER 4 YEARS OLD

Four years is a long time! Wow! I am sure you will feel the same way when your child clocks four. You will look back at various memorable moments and challenges you have had to overcome and you will be proud of yourself. Your four-year-old child is getting bigger, taller, stronger, and smarter and this will give you reasons to be delighted and make every sacrifice worthwhile. Your child will be more active now and will be mischievous here and there too. There are peculiar developmental and behavioral patterns for children when they get to this milestone. There are also issues relating to this age. Let's explore them together.

Developmental and behavioral patterns
Height and weight

According to the Centers for Disease Control and Prevention (CDC), your four-year-old boy will have an average height of 44 inches while your four-year-old girl will on average be 42.5 inches tall. Your child at this age will weigh 37.5 pound as a boy and 37 pounds as a girl. Don't forget the note of warning I have always sounded about judging your child based on averages: be more concerned with a steady growth rate. Children and adults have one thing in common: they are not the same. However, speak to your pediatrician as soon as you notice that your child has growth issues.

Language and cognitive skills

Your four-year-old will have more words to ask her questions now because of a wider vocabulary. She will be able to carry out a conversation to a reasonable extent. The tantrums will reduce at this age because your child will be able to tell you what she wants or does not want. Singing and rhyming is a common feature for kids at this milestone because of their better usage of words.

Motor skills

Kids are able to carry out hopping, kicking balls, running, swinging, and climbing with ease when they get to this age. Their muscles are stronger now and they have better control that provides the much-needed platform for such activities. Other motor skills your four-year-old child will be capable of doing include:

- ❖ Dress and undress without your help
- ❖ Pedal a tricycle
- ❖ Brush his or her teeth independently
- ❖ Walk backward and forward with ease
- ❖ Draw a circle, triangle, and square
- ❖ Draw an image of a person

- ❖ Stack ten blocks or more
- ❖ Make use of a spoon and a fork
- ❖ Stand on one foot for a while
- ❖ Perform a somersault
- ❖ Hop
- ❖ Walk up and down stairs by him or herself

Less selfish

Your four-year-old son or daughter will be able to understand the world better and a vital part of this new understanding is that your child will be less selfish. He now knows that everything will not go the way he wants and will not cry to demand everything again. He will be more willing to share his toys with other kids as he will want them to be happy just like himself. Your child will be able to recognize when his friends withdraw from him and will be more willing to make compromises to retain their love. Don't expect things to always be like this because you cant expect a four-year-old child to act like an adult. There will still be traces of selfishness and tantrums here and there, and that is why your four-year-old needs you to love him unconditionally.

Obedience

You can expect your four-year-old to be more obedient than she used to be. A vital key to this higher level of obedience is because she can now better understand what you are telling her to do.

- ❖ Issues
- ❖ Below are problems you may observe in your four-year-old:
- ❖ Unreasonably fearful, aggressive, or shy
- ❖ Unable to cope whenever you are not around
- ❖ Unable to maintain focus on a given task beyond a five-minute time span
- ❖ Consistent refusal to play with other children
- ❖ Often shows disinterest and never enjoying any activity in particular
- ❖ Not able to make eye contact with others
- ❖ Inability to respond when other people speak to him
- ❖ Issues with calling her name when required to do so
- ❖ Incapable of expressing various kinds of emotions

- ❖ Struggles with building a tower with more than eight blocks
- ❖ Cannot use a crayon
- ❖ Difficulty with eating, using the bathroom, and sleeping
- ❖ Incapable of undressing
- ❖ Challenges with brushing his or her teeth

It is important to note that some of these issues are just temporary; your child will outgrow them. However, if you notice that no change is occurring over a period of time, especially as the child clocks five, speak to your pediatrician.

Part Four

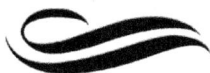

DEVELOPMENTAL STRATEGIES AND BABY VALUE

It is important to know that the potential of becoming someone great resides in every child. Parents play an important role in whether the potential of the child will be fulfilled or not. You may also ask if raising a child is solely a function of the biological father and mother, but the fact is that raising a child is not a responsibility of biological parents alone. It involves every individual who is connected to the child and takes on the responsibilities of caring for them throughout the developmental stages from infancy to adolescence and adulthood. Whatever you teach a child from inception resides with them and if adequate care is not taken, environmental influences may impede or aggravate what the child has been exposed to and this may proceed to adulthood.

Whatever you do, take a reasonable consideration of children's presence before exhibiting any behavior. Children are excellent and active learners. They pay attention even though the behaviors they have learned are inhibited because of their lack of ability to reciprocate such behaviors. A child's development takes many turns before they reach adulthood. Prof. Peter Jones of Cambridge

University proposed that the development of the brain continues beyond legal definitions of adulthood.

Children undergo stages of social development. They learn through play and in other societies, they learn by schooling. As a child grows, he begins to learn to do some things in chronological order. Children learn object representations and acquire new behaviors. Their behaviors transcend as they acquire new perspectives from others. They learn to prioritize the actions and goals they intend to carry out. This part explores the strategies that can be used in raising children of various desirable qualities.

STRATEGY OF RAISING AN INTELLIGENT CHILD

Raising a child is a process. It involves giving support and promotion of the physical, social, emotional and intellectual functioning of a child from infancy to adulthood. This process is not intricately exclusive to biological relationship alone. Common individuals involved in parenting are the biological parents but may also include the grandparents, legal guardians, other family members, government, foster care, and orphanages. In these cases, skills and strategies are important to properly raise children. If you adopt the strategies and parent your child to the social and global standard, then you can be referred to as a good parent. But failure to do what is appropriate leads to being called a bad parent and producing a child that may become a nuisance to his world, a terror to your world and a disturbance to society at large. This is as said by Jane D. Hull: At the end of the day, the most important key to a child's success is the positive involvement of parents.

Raising a happy and resilient child is not as different from you as a parent demonstrating happiness and resilience to the child. Do not forget that they are also processors of information. From a young age when they can read emotions on adults' faces, they can identify when their caretaker is happy or not. Every word, facial expression, gesture, or action on the part of parents gives a child some message about identity. But many parents do not realize what messages are being sent by their child. Resilience is the ability to withstand and cope with stressful situations with appropriate physical and psychological functioning. This positively is linked to happiness. A child's coping skills enable her to enjoy a moment-to-moment daily life. Such a child will be able to communicate appropriately, encourage you through her behaviors and withstand peer and environmental pressures.

Frank Jones said; "You can learn many things from children, but how much patience do you have?" With this, I want to put to you that what you imbue in your child is what you will definitely get. If you instill in them resilience, you give them the emotional tools and strategies that they need to solve problems and make reasonable decisions throughout their lives. Then you and they both will surely experience happiness. What can you do to cultivate resiliency in your children? Although many characteristics of naturally resilient children may be innate, there are steps parents can take to enhance the attitude in children and this can help children deal with the ups and downs in life.

Parents can foster resilience and happiness through the following techniques:

❖ Teach them to be optimistic: always make them understand that the world can be a scary place, but the child's inner strength and sense of optimism will allow her to triumph over whatever tough situation may come her way.

❖ Be empathetic when dealing with them. Reassuring words are very useful for babies to make them feel they can rely on you and others. Hugs for your kids also help them feel for others and help them gain a sense of their inner emotional control. With this, they learn to calm others and calm themselves as well.

❖ Communicate effectively. Communication is the key in every parent-child relationship. You can reinforce your child to use words like "I feel horrible," "I feel sad," and "What you did made me angry, Mom" to express their emotions rather than acting on them. This is good in the sense that, when they begin to feel upset later, they will first try this technique to take charge of their emotions and calm themselves down. Also, you should know that when a child communicates, it helps them avoid irrational and impulsive behaviors.

❖ Help them feel needed and appreciated. This is a key element in every child's survival. You should always celebrate your child while training him, as this is essential to his quality of life or happiness. When he feels needed, his self-esteem gets strengthened and he is more likely to engage in pro-social behaviors. He begins to create a link among expected actions and discriminates unexpected ones. When he feels appreciated, he gets motivated to progress positively in life and he shows appreciation and celebration of others as well.

❖ Help them to accept and learn from mistakes. If they do not learn from their mistakes, they will not be able to distinguish between right and wrong. Also, if they do not accept mistakes, they tend to be at the edge doing the same thing over and over again and make even more disgraceful mistakes.

❖ Encourage their source/island of competence. This is usually engaged in the school setting but it may not be always the case due to the variety of the children in the school. The bulk of encouragement lies with you. You should reinforce your kid's island of competence. Celebrate him and make him feel he can always do better. Use reassuring words like "You are my son, and the sky is just the beginning of what you can become."

Encourage and support your kids because they are apt to live up to what you believe of them. Lady B. Johnson.

❖ Shape your child's emotional competence. This is central within the domain of a child's resilience and happiness. Engage in using I-messages to help your child to express how she feels in statements like, "Sweetheart, I understand that you are frustrated, but you do not need to hit your head on the wall." When the child is able to label her feelings, she will be able to understand and control them in a constructive way.

❖ Get happy yourself. This can be seen as being selfish, but studies have demonstrated a significant linkage between parents who feel depressed and the incidence of depression in their children. Other studies have stated that happy parents are statistically more likely to have happy children as well. Take a step by going out with and having fun with friends each week. Laughter appears contagious, so hang out with people who are likely to be laughing themselves. Neuroscience shows that hearing another person laugh triggers some neurons in the brain that makes listeners feel like they are laughing themselves.

❖ Teach them to build relationships. This does not take a lot to do. You can begin by encouraging your kids to perform little acts of kindness. Through the relationships they build, they learn empathy and that may lead to self-improvement and confidence in your child.

❖ While you build your child up in resilience and happiness, you are definitely assured that your child will grow up to be autonomous and expressive. This will not be positive for her alone, but it will be good for you as a parent(s) as well.

STRATEGY OF RAISING A MORAL CHILD

For an average individual, living healthy is not easy in our current world. So developing a healthy lifestyle for your child is way more confusing as well. If you have tried to develop lifelong habits of eating well and exercise, then you know what effort and dedication need to go through the process. Studies have shown that many of these habits and patterns begin during childhood. Old habits die hard.

Scientists, policymakers and medical practitioners work to encourage healthy living. Although it may be difficult for you to begin to live a healthy lifestyle, as a parent, you need to do it for the well-being of your child. Remember, before your child exhibits and cultivates any behavior, he or she must first observe it in you.

The tips below are some ways to help your kids live healthy

❖ Activity tracking. Do not forget that they are active learners. It is good to track your activity and that of your child as well. The study showed that adults overestimate their activity by up to 56 minutes. In this way also, most parents miscalculate their children's activity levels, and some parents do not even know what the activity levels of their kids are. The study has also put it that while 80% of parents reported that their adolescent children got adequate physical activity, about 40% of the girls and 18% of boys get less than an hour of exercise each day.

❖ Avoid over-parenting. Do not be obsessively involved in your kid's life. Avoid arranging play-dates or stopping them from important activities as these tend to contribute to unhealthy behavior and lifestyle. Children need time and space for exploration. They need to develop an interest in their world. They want to discover and be recognized for their discoveries. Give them time to run around, play with friends and build close bonds while your duty is only to maintain and guide who they bond with and what is the appropriateness of the relationships. When they explore, you are to caution them so that their knowledge can increase and they can know what is proper to adjust to and what is not proper to adjust to.

❖ Involve your children in food preparation. Learning is a process and eventually leads to adaptation. A child learns by doing. This means if you do not engage them in what you are doing, they will never be able to do it. Make your child a doer when you are in the kitchen as this will help him to make better health choices in food too. Many parents avoid letting their children come near the kitchen, but that does them no good whatsoever. Let them stay with you and do the little dishes. There are always things a child can do at home. Apart from helping in food preparation, family dinner is another important factor in healthy eating. Avoid restricting your child's food consumption so as to allow them to make their own healthy choices.

❖ Live an example. Emphasis has always been on demonstrating to your children what you expect of them. Set a good healthy lifestyle example for your children to follow. They will model your behavior whether they are conscious or unconscious of it.

❖ Make sure your children eat at home and eat what you give them. When your children show preference for a food which you agree with over time, always make sure they get an adequate amount of it and even take some to eat while away from you as well. This will allow you to get them to love what they choose and not necessarily show interest in other people's food, which may not be good for them. Through good communication, they will be able to let you know if prefer other choices they've encountered elsewhere.

❖ Limit your child from consuming convenience foods. Limit fast food excursions to 1-2 times a week or even less. Do you want your child to live healthily? Then do not use convenience food to inconvenience your child's health. If you must buy fast food items, make sure that you compare nutrients for similar items of different goods and buy food with less salt, fat, and calories per serving. You can do this by planning ahead for meals at home. When you do this, there are numerous benefits because you tend eat together at the family dining table. Research has reported that eating together as a family helps a child in terms of better academic scores, improved social adjustment and less risk-taking behaviors. This is because your child tends to discuss their decisions when you are all together dining.

STRATEGY OF RAISING A CHILD TO RESPECT THEIR PARENTS

Research has focused on trying to give an explanation of what makes intelligence. Historically, psychological theorists have suggested that intelligence is an inherited quality formed by biology and genetics. There is also a theory that intelligence comes from the environment such as school influence, parental teachings and exposure to experiences and opportunities in life. Whatever explanation is the closest, educational influence on intelligence remains the area of most focus in research. Studies postulate that the more time spent in school by a child, the higher their IQ scores tend to be. A tactical explanation for this stems from the fact that teachers train kids to respond to questions in factual ways, solve problems and learn specific bodies of knowledge. This means that the more frequent exposure a child gets to the educational environments, the more prepared she is able to respond to intelligent taking tests and situations.

Furthermore, children who have a feeling of safety, feel well-fed and rested, are healthy and whose parents place a high value on their intellectual development will be better able to focus their attention and energy on mentally-oriented tasks and tests. But children who consistently feel afraid due to no safety, kids who are hungry, and whose parent are belligerent and negligent and do not pay attention to their education tend to have much less energy and motivation to pursue intellectual/cognitive development. Your involvement in your child's cognitive functioning and learning environment goes a long way if you want to raise an intelligent child.

These are some recommended skills in raising an intelligent child:

❖ Expose your child to diverse experiences. Do not let him miss out on things he has not been exposed to because you only cater to his interest alone. Introduce your kid to various ideas, cultures, etc. For example, expose your girls to masculine subjects like technology, engineering and mathematics. Make her understand that she can choose a career from them. Also, expose your boy to feminine subjects like childcare and nurturing, cooking etc. and finally, expose your child to different cultures so that his worldview can be broadened. Let him begin to understand issues of gender, race, and intellectualism so that he can uniquely develop his own identity.

❖ If your child develops strong interests, provide chances to develop them: enroll her in the best school which can help her develop her interest. Having your child to attend the best school possible is important in nurturing her intelligence. The school will allow your child to be amidst peers and educators who are dedicated to achieving excellence in her. Nurture your child's interests. Buy her books that she is interested in. If your child loves environmental science, find an environmental program for kids and enroll her.

❖ Enroll your child in activities that will stimulate his intelligence and thirst for knowledge. Extracurricular activities are good ways of boosting your child's intelligence and horizons at school. These activities help him develop a well-rounded life with a richer base of experience. Let him enroll in activities like athletics, debate clubs, school magazine clubs, etc.

❖ Let your child have a balanced academic life and kid-life: an overcommitted child may become overstressed and this will lead to anxiety. Because of her fixation, she might not be able to realize her potential in anything. If she is overcommitted, she may develop a loss of interest in virtually everything and this will instill resentment against her parents.

❖ Help your child develop by reinforcing his efforts and not his ability. Praising his efforts allow him to believe in himself and that motivates him to work to expand his limits in the future.

❖ Support both his intellectual and emotional needs. Do this by playing with your child. Interact with your kid as she plays. This way you will be able to learn more about her and also give you the chance of knowing the kind of intelligence she has. Do not take over her play periods. Allow her to express her own creativity. When you provide intellectual and emotional support to your child, you talk to her regularly about her interests. You will also be able to have an idea of how your child is progressing intellectually.

❖ Limit television viewing for your child. Letting him watch too much TV takes him away from doing activities that help develop his brain, like reading books, socializing and playing. Avoid letting kids spend too much time with screen devices, e.g. smartphones and tablets. This is because excessive use of these devices often leads to emotional and health issues.

❖ Encourage your child to take intellectual risks and be open to failures. Children who do not take risks and open themselves to failure such as participating in competition and losing can end up developing low self-esteem and phobia. Not taking risks may also discourage creativity and learning for themselves. Let them explore and find things out for themselves. Allow your kid to think and solve problems for themselves. When you encourage them, allow them to have an "I can do it" attitude.

❖ Work with teachers to meet your child's needs. Communicating with her teachers enables your child to get the attention she needs and she will be challenged in ways that nurture her intelligence. Talk to your child's teachers and administrators about a higher level of learning your child might be able to do outside the classroom setting.

❖ Be consistent in testing your child's abilities. This is useful because it will help you to support your argument for more advanced work and it can reveal problems such as dyslexia, ADHD and some social or emotional dysfunction.

❖ Allow boredom for your child. According to the education and training director of an independent association of prep schools, Julia Robinson, it is good for a child to get bored. He should learn to enjoy quiet time for reflection instead of making him engage in activities throughout the day. Learning to be bored is a preparation technique and part of adulthood preparation.

❖ Give your child appropriate food. Nutrition is also an essential component of developing your child's intelligence. Nutrition starts from pregnancy and continues throughout life. Protein-rich food improves attention, alertness and thought processes. Carbohydrates, vitamins and minerals fuel the brain for thinking as well, although processed carbohydrates or micronutrients have bad effects on kids' attention spans, activity level and concentration level.

❖ You need to keep your child's intellectual development in mind as he progresses in life. When you look at the issues facing the world now, whether it is climate change, terrorism, energy, and health care, these kids are the ones who have the potential to solve these problems.

STRATEGY OF RAISING A HEALTHY CHILD

The well-being of any society is a function of the moral health of its individual members. Do not forget that whatever a child will become tomorrow necessarily starts from childhood. Studies have over the years placed emphasis on the role of parents and teachers in helping to cultivate a child's moral consciousness. In whichever way, parents may also serve as teachers. This means that as a parent, you partner with children in immoral behaviors when you fail in your duty to take advantage of your child's moral moments. You fail when you fail to model positive behaviors for your children to see and imitate. Train them to pay attention and model your behaviors and you will see how far they can exhibit more excellently what you have demonstrated to them.

Do you also know that a person's sense of morality is shaped in childhood by the moral convictions, decisions and behavior of the adults around them? Your willingness to say no to a particular kind of play your child wants to engage in is a part of teaching moral lessons that will influence your child's behavior later in life. Be open to discussing the moral dilemmas that adolescents face and when you are doing this, do it in a responsible and supportive way. You should continually think about the importance of your role in your child's moral development. This is quintessential to your world, your society and your child's world.

These are active ways you can bring your child up in a morally active way in life.

- ❖ Be an involved father: research has shown that children who are close to their fathers are less likely to break the law, drop out of school, avoid risky sexual behaviors, and pursue healthy relationships. Fathers also aid their daughters in making appropriate choices among a range of options.

- ❖ Teach your child the importance of delaying impulses. It is part of morality for children to defer their impulses. They need to be able to resist the temptation of immediate rewards so that they can get greater rewards in the future. As shown in studies, delayed gratification is one of the most effective traits of successful people. Teaching your child this strategy will enable them to be patient and avoid narcissistic behavior.

❖ Help your child imagine a happy and fulfilling future. Through morality, he is able to distinguish between right or wrong when making decisions. It also helps him to know what it takes and what he must do to reach the future he envisages.

❖ Give your child the opportunity to engage in community service. You may worry that your child could fall into the wrong hands by engaging in community services. This is not true because, through community service, your child will learn core values which you may not have taught him at home. He will learn from other adults and with your help, you are able to communicate what to instill in himself and what not to absorb. Also, your child may have been brought into this world by you, but your society/community also plays an active role in his upbringing as well. So as a parent, you have to watch out for the positive behaviors and reinforce/encourage them. William Damon said that children participate in social relations very early. Their moral thoughts and feelings are inevitable consequences of the early relations and others that will show up throughout life.

❖ Encourage your child to read literature that talks about morality. An example is Erik Erikson's "Childhood and Society." Facts about morality abide around us and some individuals have taken it upon themselves to document them. Authors also suggest that discussion of such books helps to facilitate moral exploration and helps to clarify children's conception and understanding.

❖ Teach empathy. Empathy grounds morality. Train your child to have sympathy for others. Practice sympathy and compassion toward a loved one, and then to a person you do not know, and then to an enemy. Richard J. Davidson calls this compassion meditation and this helps a child to mature morally throughout life.

❖ Teach your child guilt when he/she misbehaves. If you want her to care about others, you need to teach her to feel guilt and not shame when they behave badly. Research on moral and emotional development suggests that shame develops when parents withdraw love, express anger, and exert power through punishment. This is likely to make them believe that they are bad. Fearing this, some parents fail to exercise discipline, but this can hinder the child's development of strong moral standards. The best response to misbehavior is an expression of disappointment. You should express non-approval of the behavior, why it is bad, and the effect of that behavior on others, and encourage them to behave well in future situations. This will help them learn and judge their actions, feel empathy and become responsible boys and girls.

❖ Transmit the values and ideas you hold to your child. You can tell a story, your family history and experiences to your child. Let him learn from them and also engage in the evaluation of those experiences as well. You want to bring up your child, right? Then be honest in your discussions with him. Let him know what can go wrong and why things may go wrong if he fails to respect humans or have good morals. This will serve as a bank of knowledge for your child to draw from as he transitions from childhood to adulthood and he will develop a sense of moral consciousness. On this note I will conclude with an excerpt which states:

Your child witnesses. He is an attentive witness of adult morality or lack of adult morality. He scavenges cues on how he ought to behave and find enjoyment as parents and significant adults go about their lives making choices, addressing people, giving assumptions, showing desires and values. Little do you know that you are telling them much more than you realize.

STRATEGY OF RAISING A HAPPY AND RESILIENT CHILD

According to the Child Development Institute, one of the greatest challenges modern parents face is imbuing respect in their children. To some parents, respect is not a problem they pay attention to until their children progress into adolescents. The kids often turn rebellious too. The good news is that it is not too late to instill respect in your kids before she starts experiencing tough times. Respect may mean having due regard for others' feelings or the rights of others. It involves placing value on something or someone. Children honor/respect their parents through obedience. For you and the community to benefit from your child's respect, the bulk of the work lies with you and you must carefully watch for how you can do that before they mature.

Pay attention to these facts to help you foster and develop respect in your children

Show respect for others. This is the first thing in teaching respect. You cannot offer what you do not have. What they see you do, they also do the same. If you treat people around you with respect, your kids will pick up the same habit and if you do the opposite, they will do the same. Although no parent is perfect, carefully pay attention to what your behaviors say about you.

Always speak politely to your child. Communication modeling for a child comes from home. The way you talk to him determines how he will speak to you and others too. If in the face of anger you discover that you have messed up, speaking to your child rudely, simply apologize. A mature parent apologizes and accepts the responsibility when he or she makes mistakes.

Respect their choices. Show them respect by respecting them. The saying is that respect is reciprocal, so respect your kids the same way you respect other adults. Do not try to have complete control over how your child behaves. For example, a child may love to finish eating their meat before the other food, but a parent may detest doing that because the rule is to finish the side dishes before eating the meat. This may be true, but everyone has their own preferences. Your child has her own choice, and you have your choice as well. If you do not like her choice, kindly explain the rationale behind your dislike. Always remember that kids are also humans who have to make decisions for and by themselves. Everyone has the right to think independently and have individual interests. The whole essence of this is that they begin to learn to respect other people's opinions and take them for who they are.

Pay absolute attention when listening to him. Research shows that good listening is an act of love. Drop your phone when listening to your child so that he will know you are paying attention. Make eye contact and ask questions so that he will feel respected and loved. As he progresses in life, he will emulate you when you want to speak to him as well. There are parents who never have time to listen to their kids, but I tell you, the kids will definitely reciprocate such behavior because they begin to see it as a norm. It becomes part of them over time.

Demonstrate deep manners, such as saying thank you. Appreciating them when they offer helps them to appreciate others. Teach your child to make a request rather than just talk about what he wants. Instead of him saying, "Give me more food," you can suggest that he say it in a politer way such as, "Can I have more food, please?"

Teach them to recognize people in their lives. This involves noticing what is good about individuals in your own life and discussing them in front of your children. It is excellent for developing gratitude, appreciation and respect. How your precious child turns out to be is a function of what you show her. If you want your child to treat others and you with decency, the main thing is setting the right example.

Epilogue

I am convinced that reading this book has been worth your time or else you would not have continued this far. Parenting is an exciting journey that comes with challenges which are definitely surmountable with the right knowledge and material. I am sure this material has been very helpful for you as you embark on a new phase that will either slightly or radically adjust your life. It will be pointless if you have devoted so much time, energy, and attention to this book and you did not eventually take advantage of the quality and credible information found in it.

Ensure that you remember the information you have received because any information that cannot be recalled is not beneficial. The quality of your life and parental experience is dependent on how much credible information you have and how well you utilize the information. You don't have to go with a trial and error approach. You can approach parenting like an expert when you take advantage of the knowledge and wealth of experience of others. With your attitude and devotion, which is the motivating factor that has made you read this book, I am confident you will make a good parent.

BONUS PART

Developmental milestones of children from one month to 4 years old

The early stage of life of your child is vital to the growth and development of your child. The kind of adult your child will grow into can be determined during this phase of life. Hence, it is important to know the developmental milestones across various stages of life of your child. This knowledge will help you prepare for each phase and help you report to your pediatrician on time in case of any abnormality.

One month

❖ Average weight:9.9 pounds for girls 10.9 pounds for boys
❖ The baby can see and focus on two or three objects
❖ Child can coo
❖ Child can respond to loud sound
❖ Your child also beginsto smile

Two months

- Average weight:12.3 pounds for boys and 11.3 pounds for girls
- Average Height:23 inches for boys and 22.5 inches for girls
- The child will be able to lift his or her shoulders during tummy time
- Smile and move eyes full 180 degree at this stage
- See colorful pictures
- Child will be able to listen actively
- More coordinated and less jerky movement
- The child will also be able to lift up his head while sitting

Three months

- Average weight: 14.1 pounds for boys and 12.9 pounds for girls
- Average Height: 24.2 inches for boys while that of the girls is 23.5 inches
- Laugh out loud

- ❖ Lifting up his or her hand in response to your gesture to carry him or her
- ❖ Stringing together some vowel
- ❖ Play with sensory toys
- ❖ Stop clenching his or her fist often at this stage.
- ❖ Use his arms to support him or herself as he or she raises his or her head during tummy time

Five months

- ❖ Average weight: 16.6 pounds for boys and 15.2 pounds for girls
- ❖ Distinguish between different colors
- ❖ Look at you as you move across the room with ease
- ❖ Repeat the sounds you make
- ❖ Bring his or her two hands together
- ❖ Reach out to objects with both hands to grasp them and hold them with the full use of all the fingers.
- ❖ Keep objects and show them again while playing

Six months

- ❖ Average weight: 17.1 pounds for boys and 16.1 pounds for girls
- ❖ Average height: 26.6 inches for boys and 25.9 inches for girls
- ❖ Distinguish between different tastes and have favorite food
- ❖ Examine close by objects
- ❖ Notice that the voices of people are not the same
- ❖ Say few consonants
- ❖ Hold small objects and even pull them to him or herself
- ❖ Eat solid food

Eight months

- ❖ Average weight: 19.0pounds for boys and17.5pounds for girls
- ❖ Average height: 27.8 inches for boys and 27.1inches for girls
- ❖ See things that are closer to him or her better but will be able to identify objects across the room
- ❖ Go for objects and grab them to play with them
- ❖ Sit independently

- ❖ Crouching, rolling, and twisting.
- ❖ Crawl

Ten months

- ❖ Average weight: 20.2pounds for boys and18.7pounds for girls
- ❖ Average height: 28.9 inches for boys and 28.1inches for girls
- ❖ Differentiate between your voice and others
- ❖ Able to tell when the door bell is ringing or music
- ❖ Stand
- ❖ Does not treat the fingers the same way
- ❖ Able to say 'dada" and 'mama'

One year old

- ❖ Average weight: 21.9 pounds for boys and 21.3 pounds for girls
- ❖ Average height: 29.8 inches for boys and 29.1 inches for girls
- ❖ Tantrums

- ❖ Look and listen at the same time
- ❖ Distinguish between familiar and strange faces
- ❖ Sit for long
- ❖ Walk up the stairs
- ❖ Respond to simple commands
- ❖ Feed independently

Two years old

- ❖ Average weight: 27.5 pounds for boys and26.5pounds for girls
- ❖ Average height: 34.2 inches for boys and 33.5inches for girls
- ❖ Climb onto furniture by themselves and get down
- ❖ Running
- ❖ Pull multiple toys behind while walking
- ❖ Build a "tower" of four blocks
- ❖ Use fifty to hundred words
- ❖ Child's upper second molars pull through

Three years old

- ❖ Average weight: 31.8 pounds for boys and 30.7 pounds for girls
- ❖ Average height: 37.5 inches for boys and 37.1 inches for girls
- ❖ Running and walking
- ❖ Mastery of three or four-words phrases and sentences
- ❖ Climbing stairs with minimal support and jumping
- ❖ Catch a ball as he or she extends his or her arms
- ❖ Manipulating papers and making use of tools like crayons and finger-paint
- ❖ Separation anxiety

Four years old

- ❖ Average weight: 37.5pounds for boys and 37 pounds for girls
- ❖ Average height: 44 inches for boys and 42.5inches for girls
- ❖ Carry out simple conversation
- ❖ Singing and rhyming
- ❖ Peddle a tricycle
- ❖ Brush his or her teeth independently

- ❖ Walk backward and forward with ease
- ❖ Draw a circle, triangle, and square
- ❖ Draw an image of a person
- ❖ Stack ten blocks or more
- ❖ Make use of a spoon and a fork
- ❖ Stand on one foot for a while
- ❖ Less selfish
- ❖ More Obedient

ABOUT THE AUTHOR

Mary Simmons graduated from Boston University in the faculty of social psychology and devoted herself to studying the problems of the relationship between children and adults, and has participated in research. As a member of several associations in Boston she aims at improving relations between children and has written articles on the upbringing of children in magazines and online publications. Mary has three children: 12, 5 and 2 years old. She sees her strongest achievement in sharing her own experience and skills to other people.

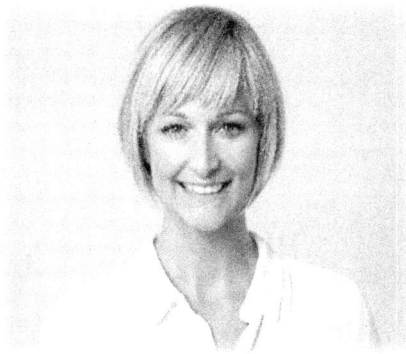

Please, Leave a Review!

I hope you enjoyed this book!

Reviews from awesome customers like you help others to feel confident about choosing this book too and navigate through their parenting times safely.

Please take a minute to share your experience!

I really appreciate it!

Here's your bonus

http://marysimmonsbook.com/home/

Printed in Great Britain
by Amazon